D1578799

Essential Contact Lens Practice

D02885

This book is dedicated to our families, for their patience and encouragement throughout

Publisher: Caroline Makepeace
Desk editor: Deena Burgess
Production controller: Chris Jarvis
Development editor: Robert Edwards
Cover designer: Alan Studholme

ESSENTIAL CONTACT LENS PRACTICE

Jane Veys

MSc MCOptom

Director of Clinical Affairs, Johnson & Johnson Vision Care Europe, Middle East and Africa

John Meyler

BSc FCOptom DipCLP

Director of Professional Affairs, Johnson & Johnson Vision Care Europe, Middle East and Africa

Ian Davies

BSc MCOptom DipCLP

Marketing Director, Johnson & Johnson Vision Care Europe, Middle East and Africa

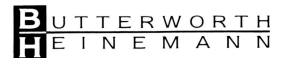

BUTTERWORTH HEINEMANN | Optician

EDINBURGH LONDON NEW YORK OXFORD
PHILADELPHIA ST LOUIS SYDNEY TORONTO

BUTTERWORTH-HEINEMANN
An imprint of Elsevier Limited

© Jane Veys, John Meyler and Ian Davies 2002

All rights reserved. No part of this publication may be reproduced, stored in a
retrieval system, or transmitted in any form or by any means, electronic,
mechanical, photocopying, recording or otherwise, without either the prior
permission of the publishers or a licence permitting restricted copying in the United
Kingdom issued by the Copyright Licensing Agency, 90 Tottenham Court Road,
London W1T 4LP. Permissions maybe sought directly from Elsevier's Health
Sciences Rights Department in Philadelphia, USA: phone: (+1) 215 238 7869, fax:
(+1) 215 238 2239, e-mail: healthpermissions@elsevier.com. You may also
complete your request on-line via the Elsevier homepage (http://www.elsevier.com),
by selecting 'Customer Support' and then 'Obtaining Permissions'.

First published 2002
  Reprinted 2003, 2004

ISBN 0 7506 4912 7

British Library Cataloguing in Publication Data
A catalogue record for this book is available from the British Library

Library of Congress Cataloging in Publication Data
A catalog record for this book is available from the Library of Congress

ELSEVIER your source for books,
journals and multimedia
in the health sciences

www.elsevierhealth.com

Data manipulation by David Gregson Associates, Beccles, Suffolk
Printed and bound in China
C/03

Contents

Acknowledgements

We would like to thank Johnson & Johnson Vision Care for supporting us with internal resource, especially secretarial support and access to journal libraries, Bill Harvey for this contribution to the CET multiple choice answers and all our colleagues who have kindly provided photographs and illustrations.

Preface

Contact lenses are one of the biggest untapped potentials in the optical industry in Europe.

The basis for successful contact lens practice lies in both an academic knowledge of the subject and a sound practical approach. While it is important to understand the theory, it is equally important to relate the theory to everyday practice.

This book has been specially designed to be practical in its approach, providing a comprehensive grounding in the fundamentals of basic contact lens practice.

The information presented in this book originally appeared as a continuing education series in the *Optician* journal authored by Ian and myself. The original series has been more recently extensively updated by John and myself and produced as an on-line continuing education course *www.optometryonline.net*.

Each chapter deals with background, instrumentation and technique and provides a summary of the topic including key points and references for additional information. The references are deliberately limited, but designed to assist any reader who may wish to expand his or her knowledge further. In addition, each chapter is concluded with a selection of multiple choice questions and answers, to support on-going professional development.

The material appearing in this book results from the extensive combined experiences of the authors in private practice, optometric education and more recently the contact lens industry. A combined tally totalling almost fifty years' experience in the field of contact lenses.

It is hoped that this text will inspire others to enjoy working in the field of contact lens practice, and to face the challenge of every

potential wearer with professionalism and enthusiasm and above all enjoyment. Contact lens wearing provides patients with all round vision, and can give them the confidence to enjoy every situation to the full. There should be great professional pride in providing this opportunity to all that are clinically suitable.

Finally, on a personal note, my biggest thanks go to my co-authors – this book has truly been a team effort. To Ian whose original ideas, motivation and action oriented approach resulted in the publication of the original series and to John whose outstanding technical knowledge, attention to detail and unfailing support permitted the updated second series and finally this book.

Jane Veys

1
Patient selection and pre-screening for contact lens wear

Increasing public awareness of contact lenses means an increasing number of patients asking for this method of vision correction. Advances in contact lens technology, materials and design mean more patients than ever can wear lenses. Perhaps the biggest factor limiting the number of contact lens wearers within Europe is the lack of recommendation by eye care professionals, even though a number of studies confirm that proactive contact lens prescribing introduces contact lens wear to patients who previously assumed they were unsuitable.[1,2] Market research continues and shows the number one concern of most patients is the perceived discomfort/fear of having a lens on the eye. The challenge facing the practitioner is to match patients' needs to available products.

Although ocular topography is rarely a barrier to modern contact lenses, ocular anomalies, pathology and patient motivation remain significant factors restricting the number of contact lens wearers. Many of the factors should, and can, be screened for at the initial fitting

Beyond the desire to increase the number of patients successfully wearing contact lenses, the practitioner has ethical and legal obligations. Patients must be offered the most suitable and safe correction for their needs and practitioners must ensure their records clearly note preassessment and baseline measurements of the contact lens wearer.

Aftercare begins before the first contact lens is placed on the eye. Patient selection and pre-screening thus become part of the aftercare process.

Instrumentation

Pre-screening contact lens wearers requires two basic techniques, observation and measurement. The key instruments, the slit-lamp and the keratometer, will be discussed in detail in Chapters 2 and 3.

A few pertinent points relating to preassessment are mentioned here.

Ideally, the slit-lamp should be fitted with an eyepiece graticule, or at least have an adjustable slit height to assist in recording both the size of lesions in the anterior segment and measurements of horizontal visible iris diameter (HVID) and pupil size. Measurement using the graticule is ideal as it is easy and accurate.

Figure 1.1 shows the preferred technique using a graticule, compared to the crude technique shown in Figure 1.2 using a hand-held ruler. Problems of parallax, vertex distance and lack of divisions on the millimetre scale reduce accuracy and reliability.

Baseline measurements and initial assessment of ocular tissue appearance can be more accurate and repeatable by using grading scales such as the CCLRU (Figure 1.3).

Consideration must also be given to the keratometer as more than an instrument solely for measuring corneal radius. The keratometer can be used to measure non-invasive break-up time (NIBUT) of the tear film, well established as a more accurate

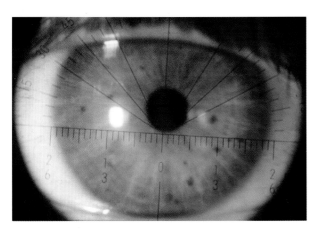

Figure 1.1
The use of the graticule on the slit-lamp eyepiece to measure the anterior segment of the eye.

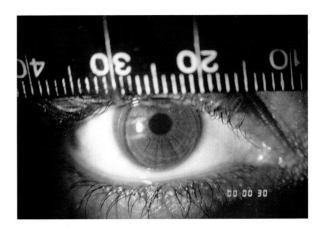

Figure 1.2
The use of a mm rule to measure the anterior segment of the eye.

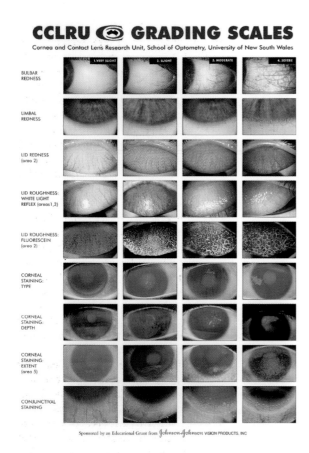

CCLRU ⬤ GRADING SCALES

Cornea and Contact Lens Research Unit, School of Optometry, University of New South Wales

Sponsored by an Educational Grant from *Johnson-Johnson* VISION PRODUCTS, INC

Figure 1.3
CCLRU photographic grading scales.

Environment	Lens type	
	Soft	**Hard**
Metal splinters	++	–
Burning grit particles	++	–
Particle contamination, moderate	+	–
Particle contamination, heavy	–	–
Strong infra-red radiation	–	?
Underwater, splashes	+	+–
Dry environments	+–	+–
Extreme cold	+	+
Solvents, gases, short exposure	++	++
Solvents, gases, long exposure	?	?
Acids, strong, splashes	++	++
Acids, weaker, splashes	++	++
Alkalis, strong, splashes	+-	?
Alkalis, weaker, splashes	+-	++

? not fully studied
++ certain protection   + makes no difference
+– possibly unfavourable   - unfavourable

Table 1.1
Influence of contact lenses in different environments (reprinted from Nilsson[3]).

record of tear film stability than the use of fluorescein.

Techniques

As in refraction, it is important that a standard routine is followed during the contact lens screening examination. Developing a routine ensures a full procedure is carried out efficiently and in a timely manner.

While there are no hard and fast rules as to the order of a routine, it is customary to start with the patient discussion before moving on to the preliminary examination.

Patient discussion

Initial discussions with the patient are arguably the single most important aspect of a preliminary examination. A correct understanding of the patient's working environment and lifestyle is important, as well as a discussion of the patient's vision requirements and expectations.

With presbyopic vision correction any option will have its limitations, so an informal discussion about patients' needs will assist in choosing the most suitable correction option. For example, the benefits of gaze independent vision offered by simultaneous vision contact lenses may outweigh any small reduction in vision clarity.

Establishing this before fitting will save both practitioner and patient considerable amounts of time and money. Each piece of information gathered at this stage should be collected with a purpose and should help the practitioner decide which contact lens is best for the patient.

Before considering individual aspects of the history and symptoms, it is worth underlining the importance of questioning technique.

Questions can be defined as 'open' or 'closed'. A closed question – for example: 'Is your general health good?' – is less likely to get a comprehensive response than an open question such as: 'Tell me about your general health.' The second question invites

the patient to divulge information, whereas a negative answer to the first requires more probing by the practitioner.

A better question would be: 'How would you describe your general health? This is important to help me decide which lenses are most suitable for your eyes.' This form of question explains why the practitioner needs the information and is more likely to prompt a full answer.

Effective communication also relies on responsive listening and appropriate body language on the part of the practitioner.

The main areas for consideration in patient discussions are:

Occupation – In some occupations contact lens wear is not allowed, in others it may be contraindicated. Occupational requirements can be found from various organizations and the prospective contact lens wearer should be made aware of any occupational restrictions.

Contact lenses may be contraindicated for patients working in dusty environments or environments in which toxic fumes are present.

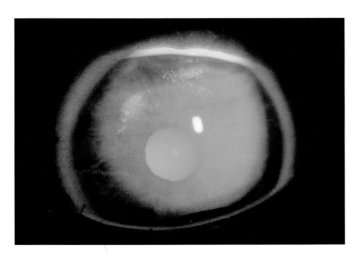

Figure 1.4
Corneal desiccation secondary to incomplete blinking.

Consideration should also be given to patients working long hours on visual display units (VDUs). Studies have shown the blink rate to reduce during VDU work, which can lead to corneal desiccation.

While VDU use is usually not a contraindication for lens wear, the practitioner will want to ensure this does not become a problem by alerting users to the importance of blinking. The use of ocular lubricants or room humidifiers may also be helpful.

Recreational activities – The desire to wear contact lenses for playing sport may be an important motivation for the potential contact lens wearer. There are certain simple points which should be taken into consideration when fitting a patient who wants to wear lenses for sport.

Soft lenses are usually the first choice for most sports and contact sports in particular. However, while all contact lenses have some protective effect on the eye, they are not as efficient as protective eyewear for some high-risk sports, such as squash.

For water sports, the patient must be made aware of the need for high levels of hygiene due to the potential for the increased risk of infection. For swimming, some authorities consider contact lenses are contraindicated because of the small but significant risk of *Acanthamoeba* infection. This risk is probably minimized with the use of one-day disposable lenses, but all patients should be informed that swimming pools, and jacuzzis in particular are higher risk environments. Contact lenses have been successfully worn for sub-aqua pursuits.[4]

There is increasing evidence to suggest that UV radiation can be harmful to ocular tissues. UV blocking contact lenses help provide protection to the cornea, lens and retina, especially against UV radiation. However, in pursuits involving exposure to high concentrations of ultraviolet light, such as skiing, the patient should be advised to wear sunglasses or goggles to offer glare protection and to prevent damage to the conjunctiva, lid margins and surrounding skin.

Patient's age – While there is no maximum age at which a patient can wear contact lenses, the practitioner has to appreciate the changes that take place in the ageing eye. The physiological changes that occur with ageing are summarized in Table 1.2. The presbyopic patient will require special management. However, the practitioner should also consider the effect changing from spectacles to contact lenses would have on all contact lens wearers. Most myopes of more than −4.00D will notice the increased accommodation and convergence needed for close work with contact lenses and should be forewarned of this.

Patient dexterity also needs to be considered, but deficiencies can often be overcome by greater attention to the teaching of patient handling techniques.

Complexion – Patients with auburn hair and freckled skin have increased corneal sensitivity. Blue-eyed and fair-skinned patients also have relatively sensitive corneas and are more likely to have problems adapting to lenses, especially rigid lenses.

Motivation – Assessment of a patient's needs and degree of motivation for contact lenses must be made. Nelson and West[7] concluded from a small study that stable, well-adjusted extroverted people were more likely to adapt to contact lenses without difficulty than anxious, introverted and less stable personalities.

Patients who are highly motivated and comply with instructions have an increased

Ocular changes	Visual performance
Decreased tonus of upper and lower eyelids	Decrease in visual acuity (reduction greater for low contrast targets and under low luminance)
Reduced palpebral aperture	Reduction in contrast sensitivity for higher spatial and temporal frequencies
Decreased lacrimal secretion	Potential reduction in stereo acuity
Reduced tear stability	Increased glare sensitivity
Cornel changes – decreased sensitivity – increased fragility	
Ocular media changes	
Decreased pupil diameter	
Effects of increased intake of systemic drugs	
Increased incidence of corneal age-related disorders	

Table 1.2
The effects of ageing on the eye (adapted from Woods[5,6]).

probability of success. Discussions should take place to allow the practitioner to assess the expectations of the patient with regard to contact lens wear.

Unrealistic expectations need to be discussed and the limitations of any chosen lens type and wear modality explained. Patient expectations are a key factor in the success or failure of contact lens wear.

Financial considerations – Practitioners should not prejudge a patient's ability to pay. The main focus should be on the prospective wearer's visual needs. The practitioner should present the most suitable lens to the patient, but it is the patient who should make a decision with regard to the financial commitment.

Never assume financial status. Patients must be made aware of the ongoing costs of contact lens wear and care.

Smoking – One study has indicated that smokers are more likely than nonsmokers to develop microbial keratitis.[8] Patients who smoke should be warned of this.

Ocular pathology – Contact lens fitting is indicated in the management of several ocular conditions – keratoconus and monocular aphakia, for example. Fitting in the presence of active pathology should never be undertaken without the prior approval of an ophthalmologist.

Dry eyes – Possibly one of the most common reasons for failure to wear contact lenses is dry eye. Much debate remains as to the best way to assess the dry eye. This will be considered in more depth in Chapter 4.

The use of specific questionnaires has received some validation in the literature and is recommended as a way of screening for potential dry-eyed patients.

One of the most established questionnaires used to aid clinical judgement is that of McMonnies.[9] This questionnaire has been modified by Guillon *et al*[10] to allow prediction of required replacement frequency for patients wearing disposable extended wear lenses.

Overall health and medications – As well as considering general health and the effects of systemic medications on overall ocular performance, practitioners should be aware of conditions and medications which may have a direct impact on a patient's ability to wear contact lenses.

Table 1.3 outlines some of these conditions and suggests management options.

Ocular history – Full consideration should be given to a patient's ocular history as well as to pathology, dry eye and motivation given the degree of ametropia.

Potential problems due to muscle imbalance should be considered, given the lack of prismatic effect (assisting or not) in contact lens correction.

Condition	Potential problem	Medication	Potential problem	Advice
Allergies	Preservative reactions Atopic reaction to deposit build-up	Antihistamines	Atopic conjunctivitis Contact lens associated papillary conjunctivitis Reduced contact lens tolerance	One-day disposable or non-preserved systems with frequent replacement lenses Monitor – check for dry eyes
Skin condition (e.g. eczema)	Excessive deposits Lid irritations Blepharitis Punctate keratitis			One-day disposable or frequent replacement lens Thin edge design Avoid contact lens wear until clear Monitor – do not fit if clinically significant
Diabetes	Reduced epithelial healing			Close monitoring
Thyroid dysfunction	Tear deficiency and poor blinking			Avoid contact lens wear
Vitamin A deficiency	Mucus deficiency deposit build-up			Monitor – possible soft frequent replacement
Systemic hypertension		ß-blockers, diuretics	Dry eye	Monitor
Psychosis	Contact lens adaptation	Psychotics	Dry eye	Monitor – contact lens wear possibly contraindicated
Hormone changes e.g. birth control Prenancy Menopause	Dry eye Corneal contour changes Changes in corneal sensitivity	Oral contraception	Dry eye	Monitor

Table 1.3

Possible effects of systemic medications and general health status on contact lens wear.

Any previous contact lens-wearing history should be fully explored, and notice taken of reasons for any past failure. Details of any previous refractive surgery should be investigated.

Patient examination

Before examining the anterior segment, the practitioner must obtain a baseline refraction and perform a binocular assessment and an ophthalmological examination of the patient's eye.

Refraction must be recorded as the ocular refraction, taken as the spectacle refraction with compensation for back vertex distance. It is important that in an astigmatic correction both meridians are treated independently in cross cylinder form.

For example:

$-5.00/-2.00 \times 180 @ 10$ mm

transposes to:

$-5.00 \times 90/-7.00 \times 180 @ 10$ mm

which from vertex correction

tables becomes:

$-4.76 \times 90/-6.54 \times 180$

and then

$-4.75/-1.75 \times 180$

This becomes particularly important in the ordering of soft toric lenses and calculation of tear film powers in rigid gas-permeable (RGP) lenses.

Anterior segment measurements

The improved accuracy of measurements with the slit-lamp graticule has already been discussed. The following measurements should be recorded:

Horizontal visible iris diameter (HVID) – The horizontal visible iris diameter underestimates the horizontal cornea by just under 1 mm. Its value lies only in ensuring that a soft lens total diameter is sufficient to maintain full corneal coverage.

Vertical palpebral aperture – The measurement of palpebral aperture is of questionable value in contact lens fitting other than in the monitoring of its size longitudinally. Of more relevance, especially for RGP and bifocal lens fitting, is the position of the lids with respect to the limbus. This can be recorded as shown in Figure 1.5.

Pupil size – Pupil size measurement allows the practitioner to predict, and manage, any likely flare from a misalignment of the pupil diameter with the back optic zone diameter of a rigid lens.

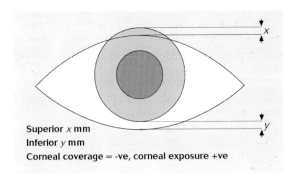

Superior x mm
Inferior y mm
Corneal coverage = -ve, corneal exposure +ve

Figure 1.5
A method of recording the position of the limbus with respect to the eyelids.

It is also an important variable in predicting rigid bifocal contact lens success. An estimation of maximum pupil diameter may be made by measuring with the Burton lamp in a darkened room.

Tear prism height – The height of the inferior tear meniscus gives a useful guide to the volume of tears on the eye. The slit-lamp graticule or slit height can be used to judge the height of the tear meniscus formed at the margin of the lower lid. A normal value would be 0.2–0.3 mm.

Keratometry – While keratometry values have no correlation to soft lens fitting performance, it is nevertheless important that these should be recorded, whatever the type of lens to be fitted.

K-readings should be monitored on a regular basis throughout the aftercare procedure. They should be compared to

Structure	Variation from the norm	Management options
Eyelashes	Blepharitis Stye	Resolve condition before fitting, be aware of atopic reactions Usually limiting – wait until cleared up
Eyelid margin	Meibomian gland dysfunction Meibomian gland cyst	Treat with hot compresses before fitting Refer for removal before fitting
Palpebral conjunctiva	Hyperaemia Follicle and/or papillae	Ascertain cause prior to fitting Depending on severity – fit with RGP lens with intensive cleaning or soft one-day disposable or frequent replacement and nonpreserved care system
Bulbar conjunctiva	Hyperaemia Pinguecula/pterygium	Ascertain cause prior to fitting Ensure minimum mechanical stimulus on area
Limbus	Vascularization	Record for baseline, if physiological loops fit as normal – if neovascularization fit higher Dk/t material and monitor closely
Cornea	Staining Opacities Oedema	Ascertain cause prior to fitting Ascertain cause, record for baseline information Fit high-Dk RGP lenses or high Dk/t hydrogel lenses

Table 1.4
Variations from the norm that need to be considered in the initial slit-lamp examination.

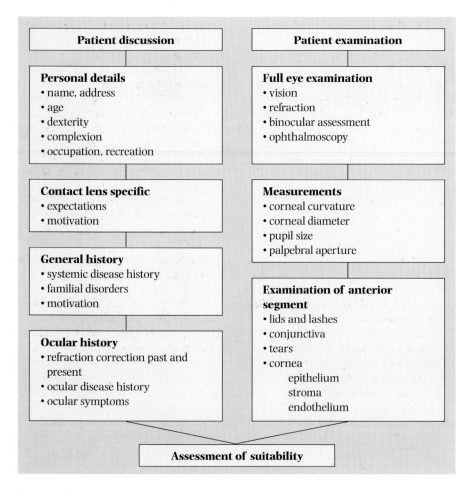

The discussion should include information on the benefits and risks of the particular wear modality and type of contact lens chosen, as well as advice on the likely ongoing maintenance costs, the importance of regular aftercare, emergency procedures and the need for patient self-monitoring. This is made easier by the use of a patient instruction book and acknowledgement form.

Key points

- 'Open' questions rather than 'closed' ones should be used to encourage each patient to provide as much information as possible.
- All aspects of the subjective and objective questioning and examination should be conducted with a clear idea of how the information will either assist in the choice of lens or help in the future monitoring of the contact lens wearer.
- Throughout the examination, the patient should be kept informed of the procedures being conducted and the reasons for any decisions. An informed patient is a better patient.

Figure 1.6
Flow chart of the preliminary contact lens examination.

baseline values taken at the initial fitting. As well as the values, the clarity of the mires must also be recorded. This gives an indication of corneal clarity and is a sensitive monitor of early corneal distortion.
Non-invasive break-up time (NIBUT)/ tear thinning time (TTT) – As well as its use in measuring corneal radius and assessing corneal contour, keratometry may also be used to measure tear film stability.

The technique involves recording the time taken for the reflected mire image (the first catoptric image) to distort (TTT) and/or break up after a blink (NIBUT). Abnormal values are those of less than 10 seconds.

The advantages of this technique, as opposed to fluorescein, are its accuracy and repeatability. Instillation of fluorescein into the eye causes disruption of the lipid layer and, as well as stimulating reflex tearing, decreases the stability of the tear film. A more comprehensive review of the practical assessment of the tear film will be given in Chapter 4.

Anterior segment examination
Chapter 2 will cover slit-lamp examination in detail. The slit-lamp examination is probably the most important procedure in both preassessment and aftercare of the contact lens wearer.

It is sufficient to stress here that a full slit-lamp examination should be conducted and the results recorded in full. Use of a grading scheme will enable the practitioner to quantify the results and should be routinely used. Table 1.4 lists the main structures to be examined. The table also suggests how variations from the norm may be considered to help the practitioner identify the most suitable lens.

Patient information

Once the decision as to the type of contact lens has been made, the practitioner must take responsibility for explaining the reasons.

Summary

Contact lens aftercare begins with the preassessment of the prospective wearer. By considering patient requirements, motivation, history and symptoms, and the physiological state of the eye as parts of a jigsaw, the practitioner can compile a picture of the best management option for an individual patient.

Time spent at this stage helps avoid unnecessary failures. Figure 1.6 is a flow chart, showing how objective and subjective findings are considered in turn to reach the final decision.

Question 1.1
Which of the following parts of, or attachments to, the slit-lamp may be used to make objective measurements?

  A   Wratten blue filter
  B   Graticule
  C   Focusing rod
  D   Neutral density fitter
  E   Joystick movement

Question 1.2
Which of the following questions is the preferred means of getting initial background information about a patient's general health?
A Is your general health good?
B Are you on any tablets or medication?
C Tell me about your general health.
D Do you have any health problems?
E Are you currently receiving treatment from a doctor?

Question 1.3
Which of the following reasons explains a cause of contact lens problems in VDU operators?
A UV radiation from the screen
B IR radiation from the screen
C Static field from the screen
D Reduced blink rate
E Reduced tear production

Question 1.4
In terms of corneal sensitivity, which of the following eye types would you expect to have most problems adapting to hard contact lens wear?
A Blue irides
B Aphakics
C Brown irides
D Hyperopes
E Presbyopes

Question 1.5
Which of the following does NOT occur in the ageing eye?
A Decreased pupil diameter
B Reduction in corneal fragility
C Decreased tonus of lower lid
D Increased corneal sensitivity
E Reduced tear stability

Question 1.6
Which of the following general health conditions and associated treatments can influence contact lens wear?
A Diabetes
B Systemic hypertension
C Eczema
D Thyroid dysfunction
E All of the above

Question 1.7
Which of the following is closest to the ocular refraction of a patient whose spectacle refraction is $-6.00/-2.25 \times 180$?
A $-5.50/-2.25 \times 180$
B $-6.00/-2.00 \times 180$
C $-5.50/-2.00 \times 180$
D $-6.50/-2.50 \times 180$
E $-5.75/-2.00 \times 180$

Question 1.8
A potential contact lens patient presents with meibomian gland dysfunction (MGD) and a pinguecula. Which of the following management options is advised?
A Refer for surgery for pinguecula and medication for the MGD before fitting
B Fit without treatment
C Fit thin soft lenses once MGD has been treated
D Do not fit lenses
E Fit large diameter RGP contact lenses

Question 1.9
Which of the following statements is false about keratometry?
A Keratometry is a good indication of hard lens base curve selection
B Keratometry is a good indication of soft lens base curve selection
C The keratometer can be used to assess tear quantity
D Keratometry measures the central of cornea
E Keratometry measurements can be recorded in mm and/or dioptres

Question 1.10
What is the preferred method for measuring the size of a corneal lesion?
A Hand-held mm rule
B Grading scale
C Slit-lamp eyepiece graticule
D Slit-lamp beam width/height adjustment
E Keratometer

References

1 Jones, L., Jones, D., Langley, C. and Houlford, M. (1996) Reactive or proactive contact lens fitting – does it make a difference? *JBCLA* **19: 2** 41–43.

2 Morgan, S.L. and Efron, N.E. (1996) The benefits of a proactive approach to contact lens fitting. *JBCLA* **19: 3** 97–101.

3 Nilsson, S.E.G. (1994) Contact lenses and the work environment. In: Ruben, M., Guillon, M., eds. *Contact Lens Practice*. Chapman & Hall Medical, 917–930.

4 Josephson, J.E. and Caffery B.C. (1991) Contact lens considerations in surface and subsurface aqueous environments. *Optom Vis Sci* **68:1** 2–11.

5 Woods, R.L. (1991) The ageing eye and contact lenses – a review of ocular characteristics. *JBCLA* **14:3** 115–127.

6 Woods, R.L. (1992) The ageing eye and contact lenses – a review of visual performance. *JBCLA* **15:1** 31–43.

7 Nelson, D.M. and West L. (1987) Adapting to lenses: the personality of success and failure. *JBCLA* **10:1** 36–37.

8 Schein, O.D. (1989) The relative risk of ulcerative keratitis among users of daily wear and extended wear soft contact lenses – a case controlled study. *N Eng J Med* **321:** 773–778.

9 McMonnies, C.W. (1986) Key questions in a dry eye history. *J Am Optom Assoc* **57:7** 512–517.

10 Guillon, M. (1992) Clinical management of regular replacement: Part I – selection of replacement frequency. *ICLC* **19: 5 and 6** 104–120.

2
Slit-lamp examination

Introduction

The slit-lamp, or biomicroscope, is probably the single most important objective instrument in contact lens practice, allowing detailed examination of the anterior segment of the eye. Slit-lamp examination is an essential aspect of pre-assessment of the potential contact lens wearer (neophyte) and in the aftercare of existing wearers.

Guidelines from professional bodies, such as the College of Optometrists (UK), specify that the contact lens practitioner must have a slit-lamp microscope.[1] The guidelines further specify that the practitioner must carry out a physical assessment of those tissues which can be affected by contact lens wear – for example, the cornea, the conjunctiva, limbus, lids and tears. The slit-lamp provides the optimum means to carry out this assessment.

Slit-lamp examination of the neophyte has two purposes – to assess the suitability of the eye for contact lenses and to provide baseline data from which any changes during the course of contact lens wear can be measured. Furthermore, in the fitting process, the slit-lamp has a role in assessing

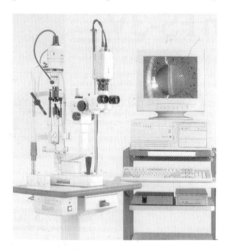

Figure 2.1
Slit-lamp with illumination system above viewing system, with image capture options (courtesy of Topcon).

the physical fit of lenses *in situ*, rigid as well as soft. In contact lens aftercare, the slit-lamp allows the practitioner to make an objective judgement of the interaction between the lens and the eye, as well as a crude assessment of lens spoilation.

It, therefore, has a role to play in all aspects of contact lens practice, and indeed routine general practice.

Instrumentation

All major instrument manufacturers produce a range of slit-lamps. While the basic principle of the biomicroscope is the same whichever model is chosen, there are several aspects to be considered in choosing a new instrument. Slit-lamps can be categorized into two broad groups – those with the illumination system above the viewing system (Figure 2.1) and those with the illumination below the viewing system (Figure 2.2). The key points to be considered in choosing a slit-lamp are:

Illumination
A bright illumination system is one of the two fundamental requirements for a slit-lamp. While halogen lamps are more expensive than tungsten systems, they provide a brighter, clearer light and should be the system of preference. There should also be a means of controlling the intensity of the light. While neutral density filters allow the investigator to reduce illuminance, they are not as flexible or as fast as a rheostat. A rheostat has the added advantage of allowing instant control which is useful in the examination of a photophobic patient.

Viewing system
The second pre-requisite for a slit-lamp is a viewing system that provides a clear image of the eye and has sufficient magnification for the practitioner to view all structures of the eye. Binocular viewing permits improved judgement of depth. The slit-lamp

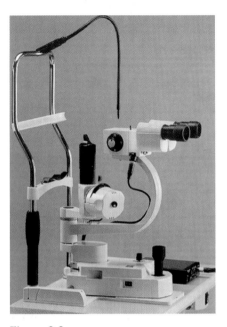

Figure 2.2
Slit-lamp with illumination system below viewing system (courtesy of Zeiss).

should be capable of a magnification up to at least 40×. This can be achieved through interchangeable eyepieces and/or variable magnification of the slit-lamp objective. Ideally, the practitioner should be able to change magnification easily giving slit-lamps with four or five different objective lenses an advantage.

Zoom systems have the added advantage of allowing the practitioner to focus on a particular structure without losing sight of it. The importance of choosing a slit-lamp with a high-quality optical system cannot be over-stressed.

Slit adjustments
The slit in the illumination system must be capable of adjustment. In most slit-lamps adjustment is variable, which is desirable. The practitioner should be able to adjust slit width and height easily without having to fumble for controls. It should also be possible to orient the slit horizontally as well as vertically. Indeed, more preferable still is

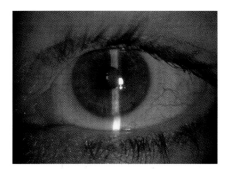

Figure 2.3(a)
Slit beam orientation at different angles: vertical.

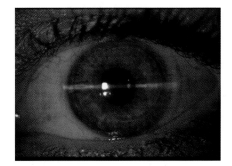

Figure 2.3(b)
Slit beam orientation at different angles: horizontal.

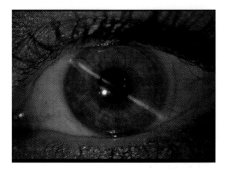

Figure 2.3(c)
Slit beam orientation at different angles: oblique.

orientation at all angles around the clock (Figure 2.3), which is especially useful with soft toric fitting and rigid alternating bifocal fitting. In slit-lamps without a graticule, the slit width should be measurable to assist in reviewing the size of any lesions observed.

Viewing accessories
The slit-lamp must have a cobalt-blue filter for fluorescein excitation. It should also have, or have a means of adding, a barrier filter to facilitate fluorescein viewing. Many slit-lamps also have a red-free filter to aid the observation of vascularization. The use of a graticule to assist in measuring the structures of the eye was covered in Chapter 1. The authors believe all slit-lamps should be fitted with a graticule.

Mounting and adjustments
The 'feel' of a slit-lamp is personal, it should be easy to use and operate. A single joystick, controlling transverse and vertical movement, assists in this process and leaves a hand free for manipulating the eye during the examination. The slit-lamp should have a locking device to hold it in position if required.

The choice of table and stand should also be considered in the selection of a particular instrument. The busy contact lens practitioner will benefit from the slit-lamp being mounted on a 'combi' unit which can easily be moved in front of the patient to carry out the examination. Tables are also available which have a common head and chin rest for both keratometer and slit-lamp – these save the practitioner time by maintaining the patient's position between examinations with each instrument.

Additional features
Slit-lamps have the facility to add on specialist attachments. These include an

applanation tonometer for measurements of intraocular pressure, a 60, 78 or 90D lens for fundus examination, a gonioscope for examination of the anterior chamber angle, a pachometer for measurement of corneal thickness and an anaesthesiometer for corneal sensitivity. There have also been major advances in recent years in video as digital image capture systems.

Photography and image capture
Slit-lamp observations can be limited by the practitioner's individual memory, consistency of grading and artistic skill during record keeping. Photography of the eye provides an alternative and accurate means of recording tissue appearance. Traditionally, the most frequently used option for image capture of the anterior segment involved the use of a photographic slit-lamp with a beam splitter attached to a 35 mm camera back.[2,3]

Conventional 35 mm photography requires a certain level of expertise to ensure the correct exposure and unfortunately the results cannot be viewed in 'real' time. Minor equipment modification produced the Polaroid option resulting in 'instant' processing but sacrificed resolution. Recent advances in video cameras, image capture boards, digital still cameras and colour printers has resulted in an affordable alternative to 35 mm photography, namely digital image capture. To create a digital image, four basic components are required:
- a system for recording the image (e.g. video camera or digital still camera).
- a system for converting the image data to a digital file (e.g. image capture board).
- a system for image storage and retrieval (e.g. CD-Rom, hard disk).
- a system for viewing the image (SVGA monitor, quality colour printer).

The major advantage of such systems is the ability to generate instantaneous images on the computer monitor following capture. Poor quality images can be deleted with ease and further images recorded until satisfied. Image resolution and colour replication are not yet equal to 35 mm photography making the more subtle tissue changes such as striae and microcysts more challenging, however, practitioners can quickly learn to capture clinically valid images that enhance patient documentation. Image quality can often be improved by using a separate background illumination source (Figure 2.4). The instant nature of digital imaging has the additional advantage of supporting patient education, for example demonstrating the benefits of disposable/frequent replacement contact lenses as well as the importance of regular aftercare. Further information on this form of image capture can be obtained from the literature.[4,5]

Technique

Setting up
A correct set-up of the biomicroscope is essential. The illumination and observation systems must be coupled and in focus for the observer, and the patient must be seated comfortably, with his or her chin in the rest, head firmly against the headrest and eye level at the centre of the vertical travel of the instrument. The stages needed to achieve this are:
Instrument focusing – using the focusing rod provided with the slit-lamp ensures a narrow slit beam is clearly in focus through each eyepiece individually, and then binocularly, through adjustment of the interpupillary distance of the instrument. Assuming only one person is using the

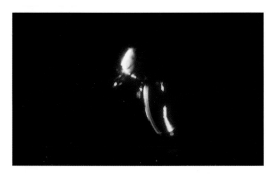

Figure 2.4(a)
Photograph taken without background illumination.

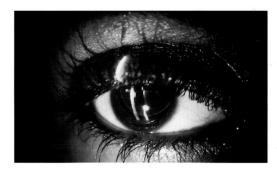

Figure 2.4(b)
Photograph taken with background illumination.

instrument, this procedure only needs repeating periodically.

Patient position – explain to the patient the nature of the examination and ensure he or she is seated comfortably. This is critical – if the patient is uncomfortable, the examination becomes significantly more difficult. Similarly, if the eye level is not in the middle of the instrument's vertical travel, the examiner will have difficulty looking at the inferior and superior parts of the eye. Most slit-lamps have a notch on the headrest which should be lined up with the outer canthus of the eye to ensure the head position is optimal.

Focusing check – with the eyelids closed the examiner should focus the light on the lids and check its focus by rotating the

Illumination	Magnification	Filters	Slit width	Structures examined	Conditions evaluated
Direct	Low	No	Wide	Lashes	Blepharitis
				Bulbar conjunctiva	Hyperaemia Pterygia Pingueculae
				Palpebral conjunctiva	Follicles Papillae Hyperaemia
	Medium/high	No	Wide	Lid margins	Meibomian glands Patency of tear ducts
				Contact lens	Fit
		No	Wide	Cornea Iris Contact lens	Opacities Naevus Surface quality Engravings Wetting
		Red-free		Limbus	Vascularization
	High	No	Narrow	Cornea	Dellen Striae Folds Depth of lesions Endothelial morphology
				Tear film	Debris
	Medium/high	Blue	Medium	Cornea Conjunctiva	Staining Staining
Indirect	Low	No	Medium	Cornea	Corneal opacities Central corneal clouding
	High	No	Narrow	Corneal epithelium	Microcysts Vacuoles
				Limbus	Vascularization

Table 2.1
Summary of structures and conditions viewed at each stage of the slit-lamp examination.

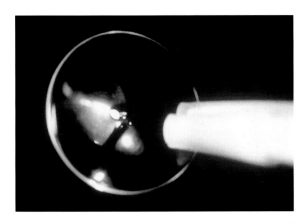

Figure 2.5
Contact lens deposits observed under dark-field illumination.

illumination system from side to side. As it rotates, the light should remain stationary on the lid. If it is showing relative movement, the instrument is not in focus.

Patient examination – the examination can now begin. The slit beam should never be left shining on the eye when the practitioner is carrying out an examination. If the practitioner is looking away from the eyepieces, the beam should be turned off or directed away from the eye. This facilitates patient comfort.

Slit-lamp routine

As with many aspects of contact lens and ocular examination the practitioner should develop a routine which enables him or her to cover all aspects of the assessments in a logical and consistent manner. Slit-lamp examination of the eye comprises several different illumination techniques. These techniques are described in detail by various authors.[6,7,8] This article describes the clinical routine in general terms. Table 2.1 summarizes the illuminations used and the structures and conditions viewed in each sweep of the eye.

The order of the examination will vary from one practitioner to the next. In general, the examination will start with low magnification and diffuse illumination for general observation, with the magnification increasing and more specific illumination techniques employed subsequently to view structures in greater detail. In slit-lamp examination of the contact lens wearer, high magnification and direct illumination must be used to check for

striae, folds and microcysts immediately after lens removal, as these may disappear with time.

Beyond this specific request, the practitioner should carry out the examination using the least invasive techniques first. In particular, fluorescein instillation and lid eversion should occur towards the end of the examination, after tear quality has been assessed, to avoid disruption to the tear film.

Overall view – low magnification, wide diffuse beam

The practitioner should carry out several sweeps across the anterior segment and adnexa with a broad beam and low magnification. Starting with the lids closed, the lid margins and lashes should be examined for signs of marginal blepharitis or styes. Next the patient should be asked to open his or her eyes, and the lid margin should be examined for patency of the tear

ducts and meibomian glands.

Once upper and lower margins have been examined, the practitioner should look at the bulbar conjunctiva to assess hyperaemia and the possible presence of a pinguecula or pterygium. This illumination should also be used to view the superior and inferior palpebral conjunctiva for hyperaemia, follicles and papillae.

This illumination would also be used to give an assessment of soft lens fit in terms of centration, movement and tightness. Diffuse illumination may also be used to assess lens spoilation by dark-field illumination. For this the lens should be removed from the eye, held in the slit beam in the plane of the headrest, and viewed under magnification through the eyepieces (Figure 2.5). Lens spoilation cannot be effectively viewed with the lens on the eye.

Corneal and limbus examinations – medium magnification, 2 mm beam

The practitioner typically starts the corneal examination by placing the slit at the limbus and, with room lights off, observing the cornea for gross opacification or central corneal clouding produced by hard lens wear. The viewing system needs to be uncoupled from the illumination system if the cornea is to be viewed under magnification by this means, although viewing with the naked eye may be sufficient.

Once the cornea has been examined by sclerotic scatter, the illumination and viewing system need to be recoupled and a series of sweeps carried out across the cornea.

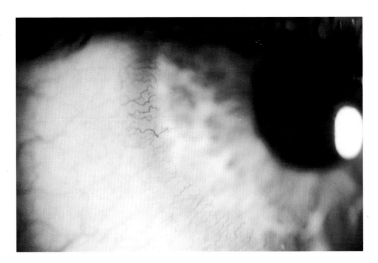

Figure 2.6
Physiological loops combined with some neovascularization.

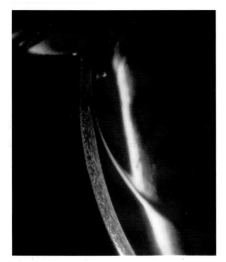

Figure 2.7
Optical section.

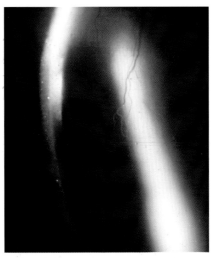

Figure 2.8
Microcysts with neovascularization.

The practitioner should start by moving around the limbus, looking at the limbal vasculature to assess the degree of physiological corneal vascularization (blood vessels overlaying clear cornea) and differentiate between that and neovascularization (new blood vessels growing into clear cornea – Figure 2.6).

Blood vessels are seen in both direct illumination, looking directly over the area of cornea illuminated, or indirect retro-illumination, looking to the side of the illuminated cornea. A red-free (green) filter aids in the detection of vascularization. As well as examining for blood vessels, the practitioner is also looking for peripheral infiltrates or dellen during this part of the examination.

Once the limbus has been assessed, the practitioner sweeps across the cornea looking for any gross abnormalities before narrowing the beam and increasing the magnification to examine the cornea in detail.

Corneal examination – high magnification, narrow beam
It is at this stage of the examination that the slit width is reduced to its minimum, allowing the practitioner to view the cornea in cross-section (Figure 2.7). With high magnification the cornea is swept systematically. A routine is essential to ensure that none of the cornea is missed. As well as looking for opacification and recording depth and location, the practitioner is also looking for microcysts, seen in retro-illumination to the side of the direct beam (Figure 2.8), stromal striae and folds in the endothelium. During the aftercare of a soft lens wearer, this process will be the first part

of the slit-lamp examination to be carried out, as signs of oedema disappear shortly after lens removal.

The final aspect of the corneal examination under white light and high magnification is observation of the endothelium. Many practitioners report this to be one of the most difficult corneal structures to examine. Even at 40× magnification, only a gross clinical judgement can be made as it is not possible to view individual cells. Furthermore, only a small area of endothelium will be seen at any one time.

The technique for viewing the endothelium involves using a slightly broadened slit beam and setting up the illumination

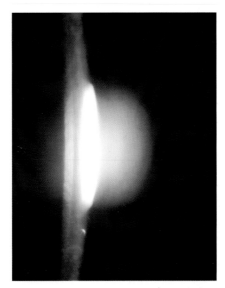

Figure 2.9
Appearance of endothelium observed at medium magnification.

system and microscope so the angle of incident light is equal to the angle of reflection.

The area of specular reflection is only visible monocularly. Focusing on the back of the corneal section, the endothelium comes into view as a patch with a dull gold appearance (Figure 2.9).[9] A clinical grade is best made by comparison with a photographic grading scale, such as that published by the Cornea and Contact Lens Research Unit (CCLRU).[10]

More detailed assessment of cell count, size, shape and density requires an additional endothelial attachment for the slit-lamp, providing magnification between 80× and 400× or, better still, a specular microscope. However, instrumentation of this nature tends to be used only for research purposes.

Fluorescein examination
The cornea must be examined following fluorescein instillation, both prior to contact lens fitting and at every aftercare appointment. Sodium fluorescein is a vital stain which colours damaged epithelial tissue. It is the best means of judging

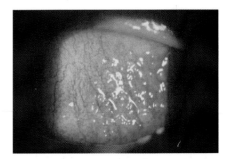

Figure 2.10(a)
CLPC viewed under white light.

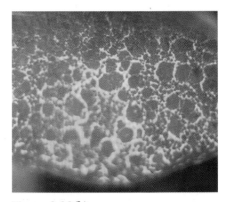

Figure 2.10(b)
CLPC viewed wtih cobalt blue light after the instillation of fluorescein.

Figure 2.11(a)

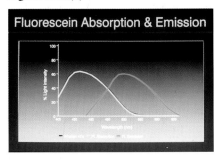

Figure 2.11(b)

Fluorescein Absorption & Emission

Figure 2.11(c)

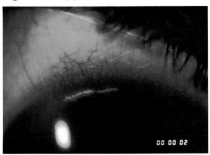

Figure 2.11(d)

Figure 2.11
Absorption and emission characteristics of fluorescein and slit-lamp photographs taken with and without barrier filters.

corneal and conjunctival integrity, and in particular can highlight tissue changes such as CLPC (Figure 2.10). Practitioners should not shy away from using fluorescein in soft lens wearers as it will reveal changes in corneal integrity which could not otherwise be seen.

Although fluorescein also has the potential to stain hydrogel material, only the minimum amount is needed in the tear film to visualize any disruption to corneal integrity. If a fluorescein-impregnated strip is first wetted with sterile saline, shaken clear of excess fluid and dabbed in the lower lid, sufficient will be introduced into the fornix. This will dissipate quickly to allow

insertion of soft lenses within 10 minutes without risk of them being stained.

Fluorescent substances absorb light at specific wavelengths and emit the absorbed energy at longer wavelengths. Fluorescein absorbs blue light in the region of 460 nm to 490 nm and emits at a high wavelength (maximum 520 nm). However, the illuminating cobalt-blue light and the emitted green light from the fluorescein must be of roughly equal intensity. The appearance of fluorescein in the eye may be enhanced by placing a yellow barrier filter over the eyepiece. This filters the blue light to make the fluorescent green stand out more clearly (Figure 2.11). Corneal staining with

fluorescein is essential and must be carried out at each appointment.

Recording results

Of equal importance to carrying out the examination is the recording of results. In law, if an action is not recorded it is deemed not to have taken place. It is not sufficient to say 'cornea clear', the practitioner must attempt to record and quantify what is seen.[11] With the graticule *in situ* some conditions can be measured, while others have to be graded using an established system. Table 2.2 lists structures and lesions that can be measured and those that need grading. Grading schemes may be quantitative, for example corneal staining (Table 2.3), or banded according to clinical judgement as used by the US Food and Drug Administration (Table 2.4).

It is not only the appearance of ocular structures that requires grading. Aspects of the contact lens must also be recorded. For example, spoilation may be classified according to Rudko[12] (Table 2.5).

Key points

- A slit-lamp with a good range of magnification and excellent optics is essential for contact lens practice.
- Establishing a routine aids a thorough and comprehensive examination of all ocular tissues.
- Use of fluorescein is essential to examine ocular integrity. An additional barrier filter will enhance observation.
- Adapting a grading system is essential for accurate and comprehensive records.

Summary

The slit-lamp examination is arguably the most important aspect of contact lens practice, both for judging the potential of a prospective lens wearer and monitoring the established wearer.

The examination must be comprehensive and objectively recorded. The practitioner should ensure the slit-lamp utilized is capable of viewing the subtle changes that may occur due to contact lens wear.

Objective measurement	Subjective grading
Microcysts (number)	Staining
Vascularization (size and position)	Follicles
Folds (number)	Papillae
Striae (number)	Hyperaemia
Pinguecula/pterygium (size)	Deposition
Opacities (size and position)	Tear film

Table 2.2
Structures and lesions requiring measurement or grading.

	Type involvement	Depth	Extent of surface
0	absent	absent	absent
1	micropunctate	superficial epithelial involvement	1 to 15%
2	macropunctate	stromal glow present within 30 seconds	16 to 30%
3	coalescent macropunctate	immediate localized stromal glow	31 to 45%
4	patch	immediate diffuse stromal glow	46% or greater

Table 2.3
CCLRU grading for corneal staining.[10]

0	Normal
1	Slight or mild changes from normal that are clinically insignificant
2	Moderate changes that may require clinical intervention
3	Severe changes that usually require clinical intervention
4	Very severe changes that require intervention, often medical

Table 2.4
FDA clinical grading.

Question 2.1
In which of the following does the biomicroscope not play a role?
- A Assessing corneal shape factor
- B Assessing hard lens fitting characteristics
- C Evaluating neovascularization
- D Judging extent of lens deposits
- E Assessing soft lens fitting characteristics

Question 2.2
Which of the following statements about the slit-lamp is true?
- A The red free enhances the contrast of corneal staining
- B The illumination and observation systems are coupled to maximize light intensity on the cornea
- C A photo-slit lamp is essential if the practitioner wants to photograph the eye
- D The illumination and observation systems are coupled to allow a three dimensional view of the eye
- E None of the above

Question 2.3
Which of the following is best visualized using high magnification direct illumination with a narrow slit beam?
- A Neovascularization
- B Striae
- C Microcysts
- D Corneal staining
- E All of the above

Question 2.4
Which of the following is best viewed using high magnification, indirect illumination and a narrow slit beam?
- A Endothelial folds
- B Microcysts
- C Polymegathism
- D Depth of corneal lesions
- E Dellen

Question 2.5
Which of the following should be recorded as a subjective grade?
- A Microcysts
- B Palpebral hyperaemia
- C Endothelial folds
- D Size of corneal opacities
- E Neovascularization

Question 2.6
Why is a yellow barrier filter recommended?
- A To be placed over the illumination system to enhance contrast when using fluorescein
- B To be placed over the observation system to enhance contrast when using fluorescein
- C To shift the wavelength of the incident light on the cornea
- D To help in assessment of neovascularization
- E To filter out reflected light of 520 nm

Question 2.7
Using the FDA grading scale, how would the SEAL in Figure 2.11(d) be graded?
- A 0
- B 1
- C 2
- D 3
- E 4

Class	Heaviness of deposit
I	Clean
II	Visible under oblique light when wet using 7× magnification
III	Visible when dry without special light, unaided eye
IV	Visible when wet or dry with the unaided eye

Class	Type of deposit
C	Crystalline
G	Granular
F	Filmy
P	Plaque

Class	Extent of deposit
a	0–25% of lens
b	25–50% of lens
c	50–70% of lens
d	75–100% of lens

Table 2.5
Lens deposit classification (from Rudko[12]*)*

Question 2.8

When should fluorescein be used?

- A At the preliminary examination and rigid lens aftercare
- B At the initial examination and all lens aftercare
- C At the initial examination and when a problem is suspected with soft lenses
- D Only with rigid lens wearers
- E Only in symptomatic contact lens wearers

Question 2.9

How can contact lens deposits best be viewed with the slit-lamp?

- A *In vivo*, direct illumination high magnification
- B *In vivo*, indirect illumination high magnification
- C By sclerotic scatter
- D *In vitro* using diffuse illumination
- E *In vitro* using an optic section

Question 2.10

Which of the following statements concerning lid eversion is false?

- A Carry out with fluorescein instilled
- B Permits detection of CLPC
- C Carry out prior to tear film assessment
- D Forms part of routine aftercare for all contact lens wearers
- E Forms part of preliminary examination

References

1 The College of Optometrists (1991) Code of ethics and guidelines for professional conduct. Section 28 – Contact Lens Fitting and Dispensing (Revised 2001).

2 Lowe, R. (1991) Clinical slit lamp photography – an update. *Clin Exp Optom* **74:4** 125–129.

3 Bowen, K.P. (1993) Slit-lamp photography. *Contact Lens Spectrum* **8:7** 27–32.

4 Meyler, J. and Burnett Hodd, N. (1998) The use of Digital Image Capture in Contact Lens Practice. *Contact Lens & Anterior Eye* **21:S** 3–11.

5 Morgan, P., Morris, T., Newell, Z., Wood, I. and Woods, C. (1997) Invasion of the Image Snatchers. *Optician* **213:5588** 24–26.

6 Jones, L., Veys, J. and Bertrand, P. (1996) Slit-lamp biomicroscopy – how to expand your routine. *Optician* **211:5542** 19–22.

7 Chauhan, K. (1999) The slit-lamp and its use. *Optician* **217:5692** 24–30.

8 Brandreth, R.H. (1978) *Clinical Slit-lamp Biomicroscopy* Blaco, San Leandro.

9 Morris, J. and Morgan, P. (1994) The cornea. Part II examination, assessment and measurement. *Optician* **207:5446** 16–21.

10 Terry, R. *et al.* (1993) The CCLRU standards for success of daily and extended wear contact lenses. *Optom Vis Sci* **70:3** 234–243.

11 Woods, R. (1989) Quantitative slit-lamp observations in contact lens practice. *BCLA Scientific Meetings* 42–45.

12 Rudko, P. (1974) A method for classifying and describing protein deposition on the hydrophilic lens. *Allergan Report Series* 94.

3
Assessment of corneal contour

Introduction

In the early days of hard lens fitting a lack of understanding of the nature of corneal contour was one of the single biggest limiting factors in comfortable contact lens wear.

Now our understanding of the nature of the corneal topography has improved. At the same time, our knowledge of the interaction between the contact lens posterior surface and corneal anterior surface has also improved, leading to advances in contact lens design.

Modern rigid gas-permeable lenses are designed with ease of fit in mind, while modern soft lens fits are largely independent of corneal curvature. These factors do not mean that assessment of corneal curvature is no longer necessary in contact lens practice. Assessment of the corneal contour is important not only in the preliminary stages of contact lens fitting, but also in the ongoing monitoring of the effects of contact lenses on the eye. Table 3.1 shows the range of corneal curvatures (K-readings) of normal populations.[1,2,3]

The most common method of measurement in contact lens practice remains keratometry, although in recent years there has been increasing use of more sophisticated videokeratoscopy. Practitioners should be aware that keratometry measurements provide only limited information about corneal contour and this should be supplemented by additional measurements and observations. Corneal size is easily estimated using a millimetre rule or a slit-lamp graticule as described in Chapter 1. A crude assessment of the overall corneal shape can also be made by judging the fluorescein patterns under a large, spherical RGP lens of known specification.

It must be remembered that the cornea is the principal refractive surface of an eye, responsible for two-thirds of the total dioptric power. Visual acuity and/or refractive correction can be significantly changed due to only relatively small changes to the corneal topography, hence the importance of using a sensitive and accurate method of measurement.

This chapter describes ways to assess corneal contour.

Keratometry – instrumentation

Keratometry works on the principle of recording the image size reflected from a known-sized object. Given the object size and distance from image to object, the radius of curvature of the cornea can be calculated. In keratometry, the object, which may be two separate mires or two points at distinct distances on a mire, reflects off a 3.2 mm central zone on the cornea (the exact distance depends on the instrument and corneal size).

The calculation of corneal radius assumes the cornea to be a sphere with a refractive index of 1.3375. Figure 3.1 shows the optical principle of keratometry. The measurement of corneal radius is made using an optical doubling system

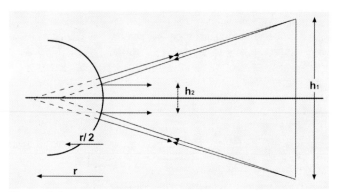

Figure 3.1
Optical principle of keratometry: h_1 = distance between mires, h_2 = image height (measured using doubling), r = corneal radius.

Race	Authors	Eyes	Horizontal			Vertical		
			Mean	SD	Range	Mean	SD	Range
Caucasian	Kiely et al 1984	196	7.79	±0.26	7.10 to 8.75	7.69	±0.28	7.06 to 8.66
	Guillon et al 1986	220	7.87	±0.25	7.14 to 8.54	7.7	±0.27	7.03 to 8.46
	Lam and Loran 1991	63	7.98	±0.21	7.10 to 8.36	8.03	±0.20	7.29 to 8.43
Oriental	Lam and Loran 1991	64	7.47	±0.24	7.21 to 8.31	7.9	±0.23	7.46 to 8.48

Table 3.1
Range of K-readings in the human population.

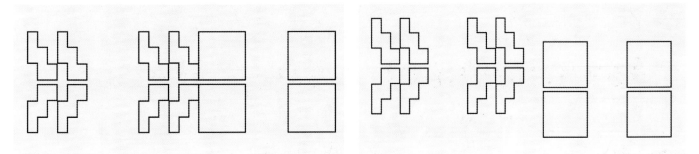

Figure 3.2(a)
Javal-Schiotz keratometer mires: mire alignment.

Figure 3.2(b)
Javal-Schiotz keratometer mires: mire misalignment and off axis.

where the observer has to align the images of the mires reflected from the cornea. The doubling may be fixed, as in the case of the Javal-Schiotz instrument, or variable, as in Bausch and Lomb type instruments.

In the fixed doubling instrument the distance between the mires (h_1 in Figure 3.1) is varied mechanically. When these are lined up (Figure 3.2), the reading is taken from a scale. With fixed doubling instruments, K-readings are taken along each meridian in two stages.

In a variable doubling instrument the object size remains constant. This is achieved using prisms in the optics of the instrument. The prisms may be arranged simultaneously to produce doubling across the two principal meridians with readings from both taken once the instrument is lined up. Figure 3.3 shows examples of the mire images in this type of keratometer. The advantage of mires in the variable doubling instrument is that they enable break-up of the tear film (from which the image is actually reflected) to be visualized more easily than the two-position instrument. It could be argued that the mires used in the variable doubling instrument make visualization of the principal meridians easier and

offer ergonomic advantages over the two-position instrument.

A final point in choosing an instrument is the way the values are displayed. In some the K-values are displayed via the eyepiece so that they may be read without removing the eye from the instrument. In others the values are on the outside of the instrument around the drums used to move the mire images. The axis can be read from either internal or external markings.

In these keratometers the observer has to align the mires manually. However, electronic keratometers are available. These are usually two-position instruments which use servomotors to drive the doubling device until alignment can be assessed optically using light-emitting and detecting diodes. The recorded measurements are printed out by the machine which will usually give a mean of three measurements and may also provide an estimate of the corneal shape by measuring corneal radius peripherally as well as centrally. Some instruments combine this facility within an autorefractor.

If the practitioner is choosing a new keratometer, consideration should also be given to the instrument table and slit-lamp. It is

possible to adapt many keratometers so that they can be used with the same chin rest as the biomicroscope with the two moved into position using a sliding table. A system of this kind has practical advantages in the consulting room.

Technique

Patient management
As with all objective assessments of the eye, the patient must be fully informed about the procedure to be carried out. In keratometry, they should be assured that nothing will touch the eye and they will be in no discomfort. They should be sitting comfortably so that fixation can be maintained with the chin in the chin rest and the forehead firmly against the head rest. The practitioner must focus the eyepiece against a plain white background before measurement can take place. If the instrument is not in focus the results will not be accurate.

Once instrument and patient are set up the patient should be asked to look at the centre of the object. If the instrument has a mirror, the patient should be asked to look at his or her own eye. It is important to check regularly that the instrument is calibrated correctly. This can be achieved using steel ball bearings which have an accuracy of +0.001 mm. Five readings of each ball should be taken and a minimum of three balls of different size should be used so a calibration line can be plotted.

If radii which are steeper or flatter than those for which the machine is calibrated are to be measured, a ± 1.25D lens will be necessary. A +1.25D lens is for measuring a steeper cornea, as is often required when measuring a keratoconic cornea, and a −1.25D is required for a flatter cornea. When using a supplementary lens, the keratometer must be calibrated using steel

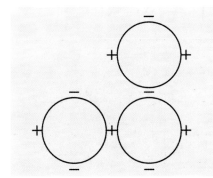 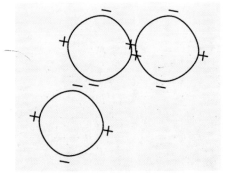

Figures 3.3(a) & 3(b)
Bausch & Lomb keratometer mires: (left) mire alignment (right) mire misalignment and off axis.

Grade 0	Clear mire image
Grade 1	Slight distortion of mires
Grade 2	Mild distortion: reading possible with some difficulty
Grade 3	Moderate distortion: reading difficult to assess
Grade 4	Gross distortion: reading impossible

Table 3.2
Grading of mire distortion.

balls and a graph plotted of actual versus recorded-scale reading. This is rarely required in routine general practice.

Measurement technique

The first stage in taking the measurement is to align the instrument along the principal meridians. The corneal radius can then be measured by adjusting the mires as shown in Figures 3.2 and 3.3. With the two-position instrument, the body of the equipment will need rotating before taking each measurement. Ideally, the reading should be taken three times and the median result used. As well as recording the keratometry readings, the practitioner should assess the clarity of the mires and record any distortion, as suggested in Table 3.2. At this stage the keratometer may be used to measure the non-invasive tear break-up time. This will be covered in Chapter 4.

Automatic keratometry

When using an automatic keratometer the patient should again be made to feel

comfortable and relaxed. The instrument usually provides a light-emitting diode for the patient to fixate. The practitioner should look at the patient's eye during the measurement process to assess fixation. Most instruments take three measurements of each eye, but it is important to look at each measurement as well as the average to check for rogue readings due to eye movements.

Peripheral K-readings

Many automatic keratometers take and record peripheral K-readings. A normal manual instrument may also be adapted to take these readings by placing four fixation lights around the object and asking the patient to view each in turn. The accuracy of this technique is limited due to the aspheric nature of the corneal surface and, indeed, to anatomical and fixation variation between patients and subsequent readings.

Keratoscopy – instrumentation

As already mentioned, the keratometer only provides an estimation of corneal curvature based on an approximate 3.2 mm cord of its surface. The keratometer assumes the cornea to be spherical, which it is not. The corneal shape is often likened to an oblate ellipse which flattens gradually towards its periphery.

The variations in curvature across the surface of the cornea can be likened to a conic section and quantified by calculating the shape factor. This is achieved by calculating measurements of the cornea at different points across its surface. The shape factor $(1 - e^2$, where e = eccentricity) varies

between 0 and 1, where 1 is a perfect sphere. The corneal shape factor of the Caucasian eye has a mean value of 0.83 ± 0.13 (range 0.21–1.20) for the flat meridians and 0.81 ± 0.16 (range 0.11–1.16) for the steep meridians.

Traditional keratometry does not provide a measurement of shape factor, so the change in contour across the whole cornea needs to be determined. The technique of keratoscopy allows the corneal contour to be assessed more comprehensively than could be done by traditional keratometry. Keratoscopy determines the anterior corneal contour by observation of a reflected image of an object.

The first keratoscope, on which modern photokeratoscopy is based, was the placido (Figure 3.4). The placido disc is a series of concentric rings which are usually luminated. The rings are projected onto the cornea and the observer looks at their reflection, the first catoptric image. The assessment of corneal topography is made by judging the regularity of the image. While this method is a simple way to make a gross assessment of any corneal irregularities, it cannot provide a detailed quantifiable assessment of the contour.

One of the earlier attempts at quantifying the corneal contour was made by Wesley-Jessen's photo electronic keratoscope (PEK). A Polaroid photograph was taken of a series of concentric rings and the diameter of each ring was then measured. From these the shape factor was calculated. Both the lack of immediacy of the measurement and problems in the reproducibility of rigid lenses ordered using the system restricted its capability.

Today, dramatic advances in computer-imaging technology have led to a resurgence in the analysis of corneal topography. Computerized corneal mapping systems have given the practitioner the means of looking at corneal contour with far more accuracy than had previously been possible.

Photokeratoscopy uses a computer-imaging system to calculate variations in contours from a series of rings projected onto the cornea. The image from the rings (Figure 3.5) is collected by a camera which sends the data for processing. The rings and camera are linked to a computer which shows the result on screen or as a colour print. Computerized photokeratoscopes use between 16 and 25 rings projected onto the cornea and allow more than 6000 data

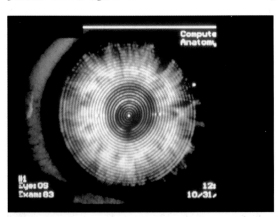

Figure 3.4
Placido rings projected onto cornea during photokeratoscopy.

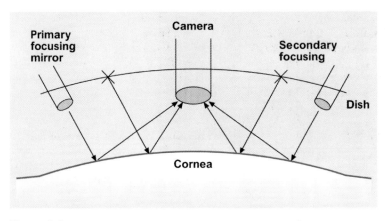

Figure 3.5
Focusing mechanism used in a photokeratoscope.

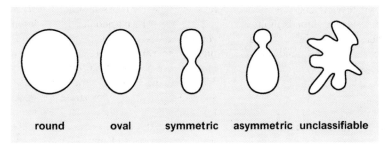

Figure 3.6
Diagrammatic patterns observed in colour-coded topographic maps as described by Brogan et al.[6]

points across the corneal surface to be analysed.

The first photokeratoscopes used a disc of 10–14 inches in diameter which projected the rings onto the cornea. Focusing was achieved using a primary focusing system where the disc was pushed forward until light was reflected from both peripheral mirrors (Figure 3.5). If light could not be focused in this way, a secondary focusing system was used in which an X was focused onto the fourth ring.

For relatively normal corneal topographies this was an accurate focusing system, although in some cases, for example post-radial keratotomy, the system was out of focus half the time. Another disadvantage of this system was that shadows from the nose or eyebrows disrupted the focusing mechanisms.

Computer-assisted videokeratography combines the principle of keratoscopy using concentric ring targets with computerized data analysis. Systems such as the TMS use a light cone system rather than a placido disc to project the rings onto the cornea. This allows a closer focusing distance and lower light intensity for the patient. A solid-state laser system focuses the instrument at the corneal apex rather than the peripheral cornea used in other models. Typically 14 000 data points are analysed with an instrument such as this.[4]

Technique

Many of the comments made about patient set-up for keratometry also apply to keratoscopy. The patient must be comfortable and relaxed when the measurement takes place and, as with keratometry, fixation is important. A measurement taken off the corneal axis may give the appearance of an early keratoconus. If such an image is seen in the absence of any other signs or symptoms, the practitioner should repeat the measurement before making a diagnosis.

Presentation of data

The presentation of data collected from photokeratoscopy is increasingly sophisticated and it would be easy to allow the impressive appearance of the output to mask the value of the data collected. The data can be presented graphically in a variety of forms, such as colour-coded power maps, photokeratoscopic images,

wire mesh models, 3D reconstruction and cross-sections are all possible.[5] The most common and useful information is a corneal contour map which shows contour changes across the surface of the cornea. Figure 3.6 provides diagrammatic representation of patterns observed in colour-coded topographic maps of normal eyes.

Corneal contour maps allow the practitioner to visualize the shape of the cornea (Figures 3.7 and 3.8) after surgery or during the development of corneal disease such as keratoconus (Figure 3.9). They also allow the practitioner to locate precisely the axis of corneal astigmatism and provide help in understanding reasons why a rigid contact lens is not fitting as expected (Figure 3.10). Information provided also includes pupil size and standard K-readings. Some instruments are fitted with software to assist in RGP lens design and fitting. These programmes will show the fluorescein fit of an RGP lens on the cornea and recommend suggested parameters. To date, the literature has been

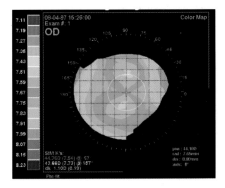

Figure 3.7
Colour-coded topographic map of a normal cornea (e = 0.45) (courtesy of David Ruston).

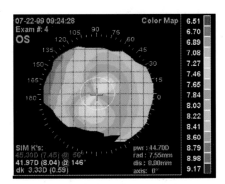

Figure 3.8
Colour-coded topographic map of a cornea exhibiting a high degree of astigmatism (courtesy of David Ruston).

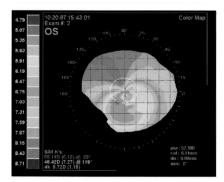

Figure 3.9
Colour-coded topographic map of a keratoconic patient (courtesy of David Ruston).

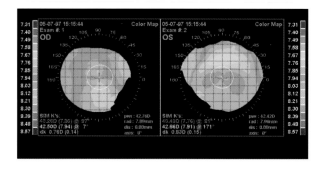

Figure 3.10
Colour-coded topographic map showing corneal distortion due to poor rigid gas-permeable fit (courtesy of David Ruston).

inconclusive in showing the value of this technique, which will be discussed in a later part of this book.

One unquestionable value of video-keratoscopy is in demonstrating to patients their corneal contour and helping explain why a particular lens fit may be taking more time or proving difficult.

Indications for keratometry

- All contact lens assessment: providing baseline and aftercare examination values of corneal curvature and any induced changes.
- All contact lens assessment: providing crude assessment of corneal distortion.
- RGP lens fitting: providing data to assist with initial lens choice.
- All contact lens fitting: determining the site of astigmatic surface.
- Measurement of non-invasive tear break-up times.
- Measurement of rigid contact lens flexure.

Indications for keratoscopy

- Understanding contours of irregular corneas to assist in contact lens fitting.
- Diagnosis and monitoring of keratoconus.
- Demonstration of corneal contour to patient to enhance information and satisfaction.
- Identification of visual axis prior to excimer laser.
- Pre-and post-operative corneal assessment before surgery.

Key points

- Keratometry and keratoscopy are important not only in helping choose the fit of a contact lens, particularly a hard lens, but more so in monitoring corneal topography during contact lens wear.

- Visual acuity and/or refractive correction can be significantly changed owing to only relatively small changes to the corneal topography, hence the importance of using a sensitive and accurate method of measurement.

- For accurate measurements instruments must be focused and calibrated on a regular basis. Patients must also be comfortable and relaxed during the assessment, to ensure steady fixation.

Summary

Understanding, measuring and monitoring corneal contour is vital in contact lens practice. Although the keratometer provides a reliable and accurate assessment of the central corneal curvature, more recent advances in keratoscopy provide much more extensive information of the corneal contour.

Question 3.1
Which of the following can the keratometer not be used for?
 A Judging the fit of a soft contact lens
 B Choosing the base curve of a RGP lens
 C Measuring a corneal curvature
 D Assessing tear film quality
 E Measuring lenticular astigmatism

Question 3.2
Which of the following instruments can provide immediate information about corneal shape factor?
 A Placido disc
 B One-position keratometer
 C Photokeratoscope
 D Two-position keratometer
 E Variable doubling keratoscopy

Question 3.3
Modern computerized videokeratoscopes typically analyse what number of data points?
 A Two
 B 3.2
 C 6 000
 D 14 000
 E 140 000

Question 3.4
Which of the following statements about the cornea is true?
 A The cornea is like an oblate ellipse, steepening towards the periphery
 B The cornea is like an oblate ellipse, flattening towards the periphery
 C The cornea is like a prolate ellipse, steepening towards the periphery
 D The cornea is like a prolate ellipse, flattening towards the periphery
 E The cornea is like an oblate sphere, steepening towards the periphery

Question 3.5
Which of the following should the practitioner do before measuring corneal radius with the keratometer?

A   Focus the instrument mires on the cornea

B   Set the objective to the patient's refractive error

C   Ensure the eyepiece is focused against a white background

D   Ensure that the patient's accommodation is relaxed

E   Check that the doubling device is zeroed

Question 3.6

Which of the following statements is true in variable doubling?

A   The distance between the object and the image is varied

B   The object size remains constant

C   The image size remains constant

D   The distance between the mires is varied

E   The subject observes multiple targets

Question 3.7

How could the practitioner measure the K-readings of an advanced keratoconic patient whose readings were off the scale?

A   Add a +1.25DS lens in front of the keratometer objective

B   Add a +2.75DS lens in front of the keratometer objective

C   Add a +0.75DS lens in front of the keratometer objective

D   Add a –1.25DS lens in front of the keratometer objective

E   Add a –1.75DS lens in front of the keratometer objective

Question 3.8

How can the peripheral corneal radius be measured?

A   Using the placido disc

B   Focusing the keratometer on the limbus

C   Taking measurements with the eye in different positions

D   Add a +0.75DS lens in front of the keratometer objective

E   Uncoupling the doubling system

Question 3.9

What is the basis of keratoscopy?

A   Peripheral keratometry readings with a moving objective

B   The placido disc

C   Laser interference assessment

D   Confocal laser measurement

E   Multiple doubling systems

Question 3.10

What is the mean shape factor for the steep meridian of caucasian eyes?

A   0

B   0.5

C   0.81

D   0.83

E   1

References

1   Kiely P.M., Smith, G., Carney, L.G. (1984) Meridional variations of corneal shape. *Am J Optom Physiol Opt* **61:** 619–626.

2   Guillon, M., Lydon, D.P.M. and Wilson, C. (1986) Corneal topography: a clinical model. *Ophthalmic Physiol Opt* **6:1** 47–56.

3   Lam, C. and Loran, D.F.C. (1991) Video-keratoscopy in contact lens practice. *JBCLA* **14:3** 109–114.

4   Fowler, C.W and Dave, T.N. (1994) Review of past and present techniques of measuring corneal topography. *Ophthalmic Physiol Opt* **14:1** 49–58.

5   Voke J. (2000) Modern keratoscopy uses and limitations. *Optometry Today* **40:9** 24–27.

6   Bogan, S.J. *et al.* (1990) Classification of normal corneal topography based on computer assisted videokeratography. *Arch Ophthalmol* **108:** 945–49.

Further reading

Klyce, M. C. (1994) Videokeratography in contact lens practice. *ICLC* **21: 9–10** 163–169.

Lester, S.F. (1994) Clinical applications of corneal topography. *ICLC* **21: 9–10** 170–174.

Stone, J. (1994) Keratometry and specialist optical instrumentation. In: Ruben, M., Guillon, M., eds. *Contact Lens Practice.* Chapman & Hall, London.

Guillon, M. and Ho, A. (1994) Photokeratoscopy. In: Ruben, M., Guillon, M., eds. *Contact Lens Practice.* Chapman & Hall, London.

Sheridan, M. (1989) Keratometry and slit-lamp biomicroscopy. In: Phillips, A.J. and Stone, J. eds. *Contact Lenses: A textbook for practitioner and student.* Butterworths, London.

4
Assessment of the tear film

Introduction

As soon as a contact lens is placed on to the eye, the lens becomes bathed in the tear film. The ability of the tear film to maintain its integrity in the presence of the lens is a fundamental prerequisite of successful contact lens wear. Deficiencies in the lens/tear interface are arguably the most common reasons for contact lens failure. The most common symptom reported by contact lens wearers is 'dryness', which implies a deficiency in the tear film.

The importance of the tear film in maintaining comfortable contact lens wear means that the contact lens practitioner must be able to assess the tears, both prior to and during contact lens wear. The purpose of this chapter is to review the clinical examination of the tear film in contact lens practice.

The normal tear film

The tear film is, typically, considered to be a three-layered structure, comprising a mucoidal basal layer, an aqueous component and a superficial lipid layer (Figure 4.1). This classic description has been challenged in recent years by the work of

Structure	Origin	Major components	Functions
Lipid layer	Meibomian glands	Cholesterol esters Ester waxes	Avoids evaporation Provides optically smooth surface
Aqueous	Lacrimal glands	Water Protein Salts	Bacteriostasis Debris flushing Maintenance of epithelial hydration
Mucus layer	Conjunctival goblet cells Glands of Moll and Krase	Glycoprotein	Renders epithelial surface hydrophilic for aqueous to wet

Table 4.1
Major components and functions of tear film layers.

Pyral, who believes the tear film is significantly thicker and has more mucus than previously thought.

Functionally, the three major components of the tear film work together to maintain the overall form. Their functions and origins are summarized in Table 4.1. It is the lipid and mucus layers that have the major influence on the quality of the tear film and the aqueous layer that provides the quality of tears needed, for example, to maintain the hydration of a soft contact lens.

The tear film is formed and maintained by blinking. As the eye closes during a blink, the lipid layer is compressed between the lid margins. The mucin, contaminated by lipid from the tear film breaking up, is moved to the upper and lower fornices from where it is excreted through the tear duct. It is replaced by a new layer, which is created by the lids pushing against the surface of the eye.

As the eye opens, a new aqueous layer is spread across the now hydrophilic epithelial surface. As it is formed, the lipid, which has been squeezed into a thick layer during lid closure, spreads out, producing a new monolayer across the aqueous to reduce tear evaporation.

The new tear film is a relatively unstable structure. Despite the presence of the lipid layer, there is still some tear evaporation that reduces the thickness of the tear film. As this occurs, lipids begin to diffuse towards the mucus. The mucus, now contaminated by the lipid, begins to lose its hydrophilicity, and the tear film begins to rupture, leading to isolated islands of tear break-up. This is the stimulus for the blink and the cycle to be repeated. Figure 4.2 summarizes the mechanism. A normal tear break-up time can be longer than the usual inter-blink period.

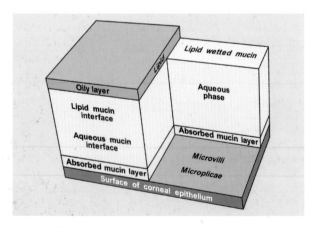

Figure 4.1
Structure of the tear film (adapted from Guillon).

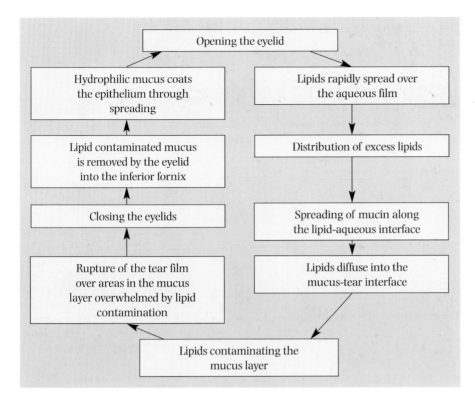

Figure 4.2
Diagrammatic representation of the mechanism of dry spot formation, according to Holly.

Under non-contact lens wearing conditions, the structure of the tear film can be affected by systemic or ocular medication, general health and a number of ocular conditions, such as keratoconjunctivitis sicca. These were covered in more depth in Chapter 1. The tears are also affected by age, with changes in both the volume of tear production and stability of the tear film.

Assessing the normal tear film is made difficult by the reflex nature of tears.

Any method to collect tears must involve some mechanical trauma to the eye that, in turn, leads to reflex tearing and to questions about how normal the sample was. For a fuller summary of the structure and biochemistry of the tear film, see the excellent reviews by Bright and Tighe[1] and Guillon.[2]

Tear films in lens wear

RGP lens wear

Inserting an RGP lens into the eye causes a major disruption to the tear film which, in turn, is the major reason for lens discomfort. Classical assessment of the non-invasive break-up time (NIBUT) of an RGP lens shows a significant decrease from the NIBUT of the tear film before lens wear to the pre-lens NIBUT. This, together with other observations, shows that it is difficult for the tear film to maintain a lipid layer over the surface. The rapid evaporation of the tears can be seen in sclerotic scatter through the biomicroscope. The situation can be made worse if the patient does not fully blink, as this prevents the whole of the lens being wetted adequately. Over time, the accumulation of deposits on the surface of an RGP lens leads to further disruption of surface quality and the thin pre-lens tear film may fail to cover the lens adequately, leading to areas of non-wetting and resulting problems.

Although higher Dk RGP materials have a reputation for providing poorer wettability, there are, in fact, very few objective clinical data to support this contention. Increasing the resilience of an RGP wetted lens might seem to lead to a reduction in wettability *in vitro*, but this has not been shown to be transferred to the *in vivo* situation.

The introduction of high Dk RGP materials in the mid-1980s was accompanied by a realization that many of the manufacturing and modification procedures that had been used for PMMA lenses could not be transferred exactly to RGP materials. Over-polishing some RGP lenses probably led to the poor wetting reputation of some of the early RGP lenses.

Soft lens wear

The insertion of a soft lens into the eye provides new challenges for the tear film. Once again, while there is a need to provide a wettable front surface, there is also a need to maintain the hydration of the lens, which may comprise as much as 70 per cent water. As with RGP lenses, NIBUT is significantly reduced over a soft lens compared with when the lens is not in place. However, investigations have shown the lipid layer is more stable over a soft lens than a rigid lens. Other work has suggested that higher water content lenses may provide a more stable tear film than lower water content products; although the question of the effect of water content as opposed to the thickness or manufacturing method remains unanswered[3].

The geometry, fit and movement of a soft lens on the eye will also influence the pre-lens tear film stability. Lenses with less movement favour the formation of a more stable pre-lens tear film.

All soft lenses dehydrate to some extent when placed on the eye, with the dehydration generally being greater as the water content increases. Lens dehydration and subjective dryness and comfort are not shown to be correlated[4]. If excessive dehydration occurs, this can manifest itself as punctate corneal staining, often in the lower quadrant of the cornea – the 'Smile' stain (Figure 4.3).

Ocular lubricants have been advocated to resolve the problem of dry eye in hydrogel lens wearers, but no one has yet shown the effect of any significant change on either the quality or the quantity of the tear film.[5]

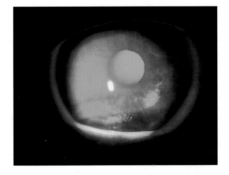

Figure 4.3
'Smile' stain.

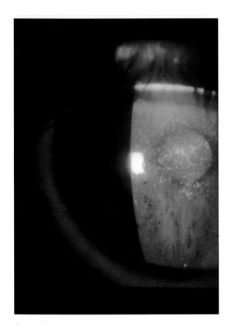

Figure 4.4
Differentiation between bright fluorescent areas of punctate stain from dark spots showing tear break-up.

Having established the characteristics of the normal tear film and the pre-lens tear film, we will now review the methods to assess these in relation to contact lens wear.

Instrumentation

Assessing the tear film can be achieved through a variety of different methods. Consistent with many aspects of contact lens practice, the slit-lamp is the key piece of instrumentation. The general use of this instrument has been discussed in Chapter 2.

High magnification and excellent optics are required to observe the structures and integrity of the tear film, using specular reflection and the interference colour phenomenon associated with them. A keratometer can also be employed to assess tear stability by observing the clarity of the mires between blinks.[6]

For detailed tear film assessment, additional equipment may be utilized with the slit-lamp, such as the tearscope. In clinical practice, existing equipment can also be modified to help to assess the tear film. The adaptation of a Keeler keratoscope to the use of the Loveridge Grid,[7] and the adaptation of a Bausch & Lomb keratometer to the use of the HIR-CAL grid,[8] are prime examples of this. Both of

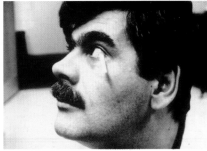

Figure 4.5
Schirmer tear test strip in use (courtesy of Jennifer Craig).

these instruments can be used to assess NIBUT.

Technique

There are numerous and varied techniques, which continue to be expanded and developed, particularly in clinical research, for assessing the tear film. In this chapter, only those techniques suitable for routine use in contact lens practice will be reviewed. Tear film evaluation can be divided into two areas – assessing tear volume or quantity and assessing tear stability or quality.

The appointment time for assessment of contact lens wearers is also an important consideration. The common symptoms of dryness and discomfort worsen with increased length of contact lens wear. Hence an appointment towards the end of the day will best identify symptomatic wearers.[9]

Tear quantity

Schirmer test
Since its introduction in 1903, the Schirmer test has been widely used in clinical practice for assessing tear production. There has been extensive criticism of the effectiveness of this technique, which has been well documented in the literature. A lack of sensitivity and repeatability limits the value of the test in clinical practice.

Although it is becoming less popular in contact lens practice, there appears to be a reluctance to discard this test, which is partly due to the fact that it is still the simplest, fastest and least expensive diagnostic test available for assessing tear production. The authors believe the only value of this test is in confirming which

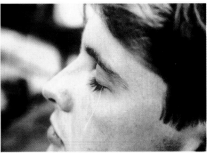

Figure 4.6
Phenol red thread in use (courtesy of Jennifer Craig).

patients have extreme dry eye. Severe keratoconjunctivitis sicca is indicated where there is less than 5 mm of wetting.

The technique involves hooking the 5 mm-folded end of an absorbent strip of paper over the margin of the lower lid. Although variations have been produced, the most commonly used is the Schirmer tear test strip, which comprises absorbent strips of paper of 35 mm × 5 mm (Figure 4.5). The length of the wetting from the bend is measured in millimetres after five minutes. A normal tear film should produce a wetting length of more than 15 mm.

Phenol red thread test
This method of assessing tear quantity has the advantage of being less invasive than the Schirmer test, utilizing a two-ply cotton thread impregnated with phenol red dye (Figure 4.6). Phenol red is pH sensitive and changes from yellow to red when wetted by tears.

To undertake this test, the crimped end of a 70 mm long thread is placed in the inferior conjunctival sac on the temporal side. The patient is instructed to close his or her eyes and the thread is removed after 15 seconds. The length of the colour change on the thread – indicating the length of the thread wetted by the tears – is measured in millimetres. Wetting lengths should normally be between 9 mm and 20 mm. Values of less than 9 mm have been shown to correlate with subjective symptoms of dryness.

Inferior tear prism height
Measuring the tear meniscus formed on the lower lid margins gives a useful guide to tear volume. The authors believe this test should be an integral part of the pre-assessment of potential contact lens wearers. This simple technique employs the slit-lamp biomicro-

scope. Excessive or prolonged use of illumination should be avoided to prevent artificial drying of the tear prism. With experience, the approximate prism is graded as minimal, normal or excessive. Grading is not accurate in the presence of reflex tearing.

Figure 4.7 shows the appearance of the tear prism through a slit-lamp. For precise measurement, a graticule can be employed in the slit-lamp eyepiece.

An alternative technique is to compare the tear prism height with the illuminated slit width by setting the slit horizontally in alignment with the lower lid margin; the slit width is altered until it appears to match the height of the tear prism. A value in millimetres can be obtained by a one-off calibration of the knob rotation controlling the slit width, using a microscope scale.

Guillon proposes a clinical routine to incorporate the measurement of the tear film prism height in these positions:
• Immediately below the pupil centre
• 5 mm nasally
• 5 mm temporally

This approach allows the evaluation of the regularity, in addition to the volume, of the tear film. Figure 4.8 shows the normal distribution of tear prism heights, peaking at 0.22 mm.[10] It is important to ensure that the patient is in the primary position of gaze, as the apparent height of the meniscus can depend on the position of gaze.

Tear quality

The difficulty in assessing the quality of the tear film is in developing a system to observe accurately a transparent structure.

Fluorescein BUT
Traditionally, tear break-up time has been measured by staining the tears with fluorescein to assist with observing and viewing the dyed tear film under cobalt blue light. The dye is usually applied by wetting a fluorescein-impregnated strip with saline, then shaking off any excess liquid and gently touching the lower conjunctiva with the strip tip. Alternatively, a drop of a 1 per cent or 2 per cent fluorescein solution from a Minim can be instilled directly into the lower fornix. A BUT of 20 seconds is considered a normal value for tear film stability, although wide ranges have been reported in the literature.

It should be noted that this technique is invasive. Touching the eye with the paper strip will induce a degree of reflex tearing and instilling 20–30 ml of fluorescein solution from a Minim swamps the normal 7 ml tear film. Furthermore, the addition of fluorescein to the tear film alters the physical interactions between the tear film layers, which reduces the surface tension and, hence, affects the BUT value. It should also be remembered that the fluorescein dye stains soft lenses and this precludes its use in assessing the pre-lens tear film with a soft lens *in situ*.

Practitioners should be aware of all these limitations and, therefore, consider other, more reliable and non-invasive options for assessing tear stability.

Non-invasive break-up time
This is the measurement, in seconds, of the time that elapses between the last complete blink and the appearance of the first discontinuity in the tear film. A pre-rupture phase, known as the tear thinning time (TTT), can also be observed with some techniques. A number of different instruments can be employed to measure NIBUT. A summary of those that are suitable for use in routine contact lens practice is given in Table 4.2. All techniques listed can be used with and without contact lenses.

All these methods are optical in nature and measurement is achieved by observing the distortion (TTT) and/or break up (NIBUT) of a keratometer mire, the reflected grid image or changing interference patterns. The practitioner views the first Purkinje image and records the time taken for the image to distort and/or break up. Figures 4.9 and 4.10 show the reflected images from the HIR-CAL grid.

Well-documented research papers confirm that NIBUT is, typically, longer than fluorescein BUT, and is often greater than 30 seconds (Figure 4.11). Abnormal values are those of less than 15 seconds. These methods are considered to be more patient-friendly and, furthermore, more repeatable and precise. As with most clinical methods of tear assessment, measurements are not reliable if reflex tearing is observed.

Specular reflection observation
This is a method for observing the tear film in specular reflection that does not require the instillation of a dye. Two techniques can be employed in clinical practice.

Narrow-field specular reflection
The bright reflection from the slit beam is

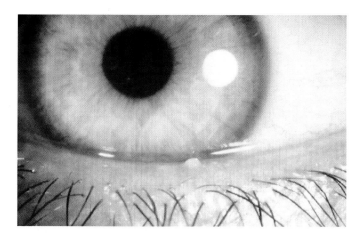

Figure 4.7
Inferior tear prism as seen with the slit-lamp biomicroscope.

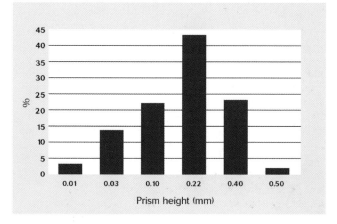

Figure 4.8
Inferior prism height distribution.[10]

Instrument	Target	Background	Additional comments	Author
Keratometer	Mire	Dark field	Only shows reflected disturbances on 3mm circumference	Patel 1985
Modified keratometer	HIR-CAL grid	Dark field	Normal use of keratometer restricted	Hirji *et al* 1989
Hand-held keratoscope	Loveridge grid	Dark field		Loveridge 1993
Tearscope		White field	Also allows evaluation of tear structure	Guillon 1986

Table 4.2
Techniques to measure NIBUT.

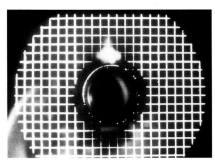

Figure 4.9
Undistorted reflected image from the HIR-CAL grid (courtesy of Sudi Patel).

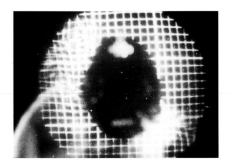

Figure 4.10
Distorted reflected image from the HIR-CAL grid (courtesy of Sudi Patel).

located and brought into focus through a slit lamp utilizing high magnification (30-40×). It is important to reduce the light intensity to avoid artificially drying the tear film and to subtend as large an angle as possible with the light source. Although it is a relatively easy technique to undertake, its greatest limitation is that it permits only a very small area to be observed at any one time (1 mm × 2 mm-zone maximum).

Tearscope

This is a hand-held instrument that is

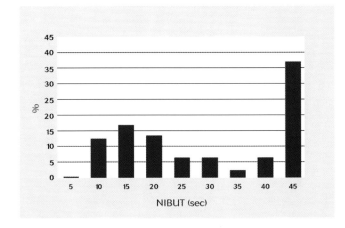

Figure 4.11
NIBUT distribution.

designed to be used in conjunction with a slit-lamp biomicroscope. The Tearscope (Keeler Ltd), developed by Guillon in 1986, comprises a 90 mm hemispherical cup and handle with a central 15 mm diameter observation hole. The inner cup surface is illuminated by a cold cathode ring light source, which is specifically designed to prevent any artificial drying of the tear film during an examination. The light emitted is diffuse and, as such, does not need to be in focus to observe the tear film.

With the patient's head positioned on the slit-lamp chin rest, the slit-lamp source should be positioned nasally and switched off. Alternative illumination is provided by the Tearscope itself. The Tearscope should then be held as close to the eye as possible and positioned to allow observation through the sight hole via one of the biomicroscope objectives. The closer the Tearscope is to the eye the better, so that the area illuminated can be maximized. The light reflected from the tear film can be

observed as a white circular area, 10–12 mm in diameter. Initially, set the magnification on low, although this can be increased up to 20–40× to examine the interference patterns in detail.

This device allows both the measurement

Key points

- Tear film assessment should be undertaken with minimal invasion of the structure – non-invasive techniques should be used whenever possible.
- Assessment must be made both prior to and during the contact lens wear. Tear film quality should be assessed both with the lens *in situ* and without the lens.
- Using the Tearscope allows a more detailed examination of the tears to be undertaken.

Description	Incidence (%)	Estimated thickness (nm)	Appearance	Clinical
Open marmoreal	21	15	Grey, marble-like open meshwork pattern	Contact lens drying problems
Closed marmoreal	10	30	Grey, marble-like tight meshwork pattern	Stable tear film Good contact lens candidate
Flow	23	30–80	Wavy, constantly changing round shape	Generally stable tear film. Possible contact lens candidate. Possible excess lipid deposition
Amorphous	24	80	Blue/white appearance	Highly stable tear film. Excellent contact lens candidate. Occasional greasing problems
Colour	15	80–370	Yellow, brown, blue and purple fringes grey background	Contact lens wear possible but excessive lipid deposition likely
Other	7	Variable	Variable coloured fringes with mucus strands	Contact lens wear contraindicated

Table 4.3
Lipid pattern classification, incidence and clinical interpretation, adapted from Guillon and Guillon.[10]

of the non-invasive break-up time and the assessment of the lipid layer. Interpreting the interference patterns observed takes time to perfect, but excellent video training material is available. Figure 4.12 displays the patterns typically seen in the normal population. Table 4.3 outlines the classification, incidence and clinical interpretation of the various patterns.

Of course, comprehensive tear film assessment is not a stand-alone examination. Importantly, all adjacent structures should be evaluated. This assessment should be undertaken using a slit-lamp and diffuse illumination. Lashes, lid margins, the inner and outer canthus and meibomian glands should all be examined. Traces of make-up and blepharitis, among others, will impact on the tear film.

Furthermore, careful questioning of the patient provides important information in evaluating the tear film (see Chapter 1). Using specific questionnaires to aid clinical judgement can be of benefit. Readers should see the most established questionnaire by McMonnies – an excellent method of screening for dry-eye patients.[11] This questionnaire divides symptoms into primary/non-provoked (e.g. soreness, grittiness) and secondary/provoked (e.g. irritation from smoke, chlorine), and provides a score for a subject's potential for contact lens tolerance/non-tolerance.

Summary

The examination of the tear film is one of the most important aspects of assessing potential contact lens wearers and the

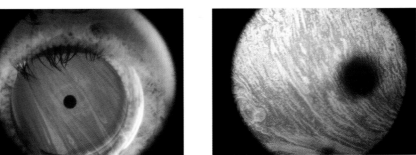

Figure 4.12
Typical patterns seen through a Tearscope: meshwork and waves (left), waves (centre), colour fringes (right) (courtesy of Contact Lens Research Consultants, London).

aftercare of existing patients. The very nature of contact lens wear results in a tear film that is thinner and less stable than the pre-ocular tear film. The transparency of the tears makes them difficult to examine, and the challenge to the practitioner is in developing a technique to visualize the structure without causing disruption.

The use of fluorescein and Schirmer strips as the standard means of assessment has been superseded by non-invasive techniques that increase the accuracy of the investigation. Consideration of patient symptoms is also critical in the overall clinical assessment.

Question 4.1

The tear compound which enables the tears to wet the normal epithelium is:
  A Secreted from the meibomian glands
  B A glycoprotein layer on the anterior surface of the tears
  C Produced from the glands of Moll and Krause
  D An ester wax
  E Provides an optically smooth surface

Question 4.2

The stimulus for blinking and replenishment of the tear film is:
  A Excess lipid distribution in the inferior fornix
  B Loss of hydrophilicity of the mucus contaminated by lipid
  C Excess mucus accumulation in the inferior fornix
  D Evaporation of the surface lipid layer
  E Contamination of the lipid layer with glycoproteins

Question 4.3

The tear film of an RGP wearer:
  A Has a decreased NIBUT in comparison to a non-wearer
  B Has a thicker lipid layer than a non-wearer
  C Has a more stable lipid layer than a non-contact lens wearer
  D Contains no mucus layer
  E Maintains its stability through producing more aqueous layer

Question 4.4

The tear film of a soft lens wearer is not influenced by:
  A Water content
  B Lens movement
  C Lens thickness
  D Ocular lubricant
  E Lens deposition

Question 4.5

Which of the following provides an assessment of tear quantity?
  A HIR-CAL grid
  B Assessment of keratometry image
  C Inferior tear prism height
  D Loveridge grid
  E Specular reflection

Question 4.6

Which of the following is true?
  A The Loveridge grid fits on to the keratometer and assesses tear quality
  B The Tearscope provides a means of assessing tear production
  C NIBUT values obtained with the HIR-CAL are greater than those found with fluorescein
  D NIBUT values obtained with the HIR-CAL are less than those found with fluorescein
  E The HIR-CAL grid can also be used for assessing corneal radius

Question 4.7

Which of the following tear patterns is most likely to be associated with contact lens drying problems?
  A Closed marmoreal
  B Stable amorphous
  C Open marmoreal
  D Trace colour fringes
  E Flow

Question 4.8

Which of the following statements about the Tearscope is FALSE?
  A Is the only way to visualize the relative thickness of the tear film
  B Should be used with a biomicroscope
  C Provides an assessment of NIBUT
  D Assesses tear quality
  E Allows assessment of the lipid layer

Question 4.9

What is the major advantage of measuring NIBUT?
  A It can be carried out at the same time as keratometry
  B It gives information about tear quality, as well as quantity
  C It assesses a larger area of the tear film
  D The tear film is examined in a more natural state
  E Tear film evaporation is minimal

Question 4.10

Compared to pre-ocular tear film, the pre-lens tear film is:
  A Thicker
  B More stable
  C Same thickness
  D Thinner
  E More easily observed

References

1 Bright, A.M. and Tighe, B.J. (1993) The composition and interfacial properties of tears, tear substitutes and tear models. *JBCLA* **16:2** 57–66.
2 Guillon, J.P. (1986) Tear film structure and contact lenses. In: Holly, F.J., ed. The Preocular Tear Film in Health, Disease and Contact Lens Wear. **85:** 815–939. Dry Eye Institute.
3 Young, G. and Efron, N. (1991) Characteristics of the pre-lens tear film during hydrogel contact lens wear. *Ophthalmic Physiol Opt* **11:1** 53–58.
4 Fonn, D. and Simpson, T. (1999) Hydrogel lens dehydration and subjective comfort and dryness ratings in symptomatic and asymptomatic contact lens wearers. *Optom Vis Sci* **76:10** 700–704.
5 Efron, N. (1990) Do in-eye lubricants for contact lens wearers really work? *Trans BCLA* 14–19.
6 Patel, S. (1985) Effects of fluorescein on tear break-up time and on tear timing time. *Am J Optom Physiol Opt* **62:3** 188–190.
7 Loveridge, R. (1993) Breaking up is hard to do? **33:21** *Optometry Today* 18–24.
8 Hirji, N., Patel, S. and Callender, M. (1989) Human tear film pre-rupture phase time (TP-RPT): a non-invasive technique for evaluating the pre-corneal tear film using a novel keratometer wire. *Ophthalmic Physiol Opt* **9:4** 139–142.
9 Begley, C. (2000) Responses of contact lens wearers to a dry eye survey. *Optom Vis Sci* **77:1** 40–46.
10 Guillon, J.P. and Guillon, M. (1994) The role of tears in contact lens performance and its measurement. In: Ruben, M. and Guillon, M. eds. *Contact Lens Practice.* Chapman and Hall Medical, Chapter 21 453–483.
11 McMonnies, C. (1986) Key questions in a dry-eye history. *J Am Optom Assoc* **57:7** 512–517.

5
Soft contact lens fitting

Introduction

It has been argued that the skill in contact lens practice has moved away from the mechanics of lens fitting to monitoring the ocular physiology of the patient. Nowhere is this truer than in soft lens fitting, in which the options available to the practitioner are often limited to a 'one-fit' lens design. Despite this change in the availability of lens designs, most contact lens teaching is still based on practitioners having a number of different designs available.

Many of the myths surrounding soft contact lens fitting and design have been summarized in the literature.[1] The purpose of this chapter is to provide a practical overview of the key aspects of soft contact lens fitting principles and not to deal with specific products.

The ideal soft contact lens fit

Judging the fit involves evaluating both static and dynamic criteria. The ideal soft contact lens fit should show the following characteristics:

Corneal coverage
The lens should cover the cornea in primary gaze at all times, as shown in Figure 5.1. This is to avoid desiccation of an exposed cornea, leading to epithelial staining.

Dynamic fit
The lens must allow tear exchange to enable metabolic debris from the cornea to be excreted. It is now well established that soft contact lens movement plays only a minor role in corneal oxygenation.

Figure 5.2 shows a comparison of the tear pump effect of a soft versus a hard lens. This is more significant for managing the soft contact lens patient. The practitioner should not increase lens movement to alleviate hypoxic signs in the soft lens wearer. This will be covered in more detail in a later part of this chapter.

Alignment
The lens should align with the cornea and the conjunctiva and should show no indentation of conjunctival vessels that would indicate stagnation of tears in this region and reduced oxygen supply to the limbus. The lens should also show no edge stand-off that would lead to discomfort and, possibly, excessive movement.

Lens centration
The lens should remain approximately central to the cornea in all positions of gaze. A failure to achieve this will result in episodes of corneal desiccation and mechanical stress on the peripheral cornea.

Patient response
When the above four criteria are attained, the patient should achieve comfort and crisp stable vision with the lens. As a general guide, comfort and subjective vision should be graded as eight or more out of ten for a satisfactory response.

Instrumentation – keratometry

Trial lens selection
Keratometry readings are a poor indication of soft lens fit, and several studies, such as

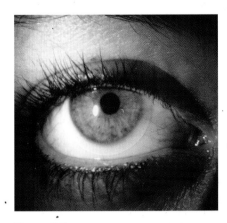

Figure 5.1
Lens fit in primary position of gaze.

Gundal,[2] have shown no correlation between either central or peripheral K-readings and the best-fitting soft contact lens. Despite this, fitting guides continue to be produced in which K-readings are quoted as being measurements on which the initial base curve is selected.

The reason why K-readings do not predict a soft lens fit has been explained by Young.[3] The relationship between the sagittal height (sag) of the lens and the sag of the anterior segment of the eye over the lens diameter determines the fit of the lens.

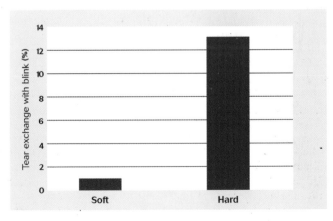

Figure 5.2
The effect of the tear pump with contact lens wear.

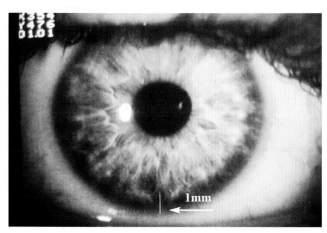

Figure 5.3(a)
Superimposed measurement cursor illustrating 1 mm.

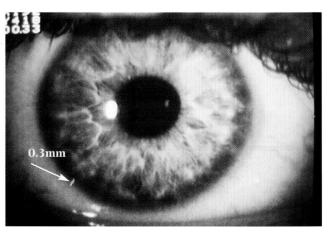

Figure 5.3(b)
Superimposed measurement cursor illustrating 0.3 mm.

If the lens sag is greater than the ocular sag, then the lens will fit steeply, and vice versa. By using a mathematical model to calculate ocular sag and then inputting normal ranges of values for each variable with the model, Young showed that the normal population variability in shape factor had a greater effect on sag than either corneal radius or diameter.

Keratometry does not play a role in the selection of the initial trial lens. The keratometer should not, however, be ignored in soft lens fitting.

Baseline data
As was mentioned earlier in this book, baseline keratometry readings should be taken for comparative purposes.

Tear quality
The keratometer can be used to measure the pre-lens tear break-up time to indicate a potential dry-eye problem during fitting.

Judging lens fit
The quality of the keratometer mires pre and post blink can be used to help to judge the fitting characteristics. The mires should remain clear at all stages. With a steep fitting lens, the mires will look blurred prior to a blink and clear post blink, and, with a loose fitting lens, the converse will occur. While this is often cited as a method for judging the lens fit, the authors believe this method has limited application to modern thin lens designs.

Corneal topography
Corneal topography can be used to locate the apex of the cornea. This is valuable because the lens will centre on the corneal apex rather than on the geometric centre of the cornea. If the apex is displaced, the lens will decentre. Locating the apex will help in determining the best management option to overcome it.

Retinoscopy

The retinoscope can be used in the same way as judging keratometer mire quality to assess lens fit. The goal is to have a crisp, clear and stable image at all times. Variation from this indicates that the lens fit is sub-optimal. This could be used as a relatively crude check of the lens fit prior to a more detailed analysis. It will, however, give a good indication of the reasons why a patient's vision does not meet the required standard. The retinoscope can play a useful role in domiciliary visits if there is a need to fit a bandage lens.

PD rule

The normal PD rule may be used for measuring gross external parameters. Horizontal visible iris diameter (HVID) can be measured and is of value to the soft lens fitting as it will act as a determinant of total diameter. As a guide, the HVID must be at least 1 mm less than the total diameter (TD) of the lens to be fitted. However, without this measurement soft lens assessment on the eye will quickly determine whether the lens TD is suitable. In addition, measuring the anterior segment by using such a PD rule is a crude method, so utilizing a graticule on the slit lamp should be encouraged.

Biomicroscopy

As in so many aspects of contact lens practice, the biomicroscope is an essential tool. In soft lens fitting, its primary purpose is to allow the practitioner to judge and then record the fit of the lens on the eye. The basic use of the slit-lamp has already been covered in Chapter 2, which discussed the attributes that a slit-lamp should have.

The importance of a graticule in a slit-lamp for recording lesions and for anterior segment measurements has already been discussed in Chapter 1. In soft lens fitting, the graticule also allows the practitioner to assess accurately the precise post-blink measurement of a contact lens.

While many texts and fitting guides still refer to an optimally fitting soft contact lens as being 1 mm, the actual post-blink movement usually measures 0.2 mm to 0.4 mm.

In Figure 5.3(a), a cursor is superimposed on the eye to demonstrate just how 'big' 1 mm looks through a slit-lamp. A lens that moves as much as the marker does in Figure 5.3(a) would be judged by most practitioners as showing excessive movement, even though the recorded measurement is 1 mm. In fact, the amount shown in Figure 5.3(b) is closer to that typically seen in a soft contact lens and, in this case, is 0.3 mm.

As well as recording lens movement, the slit-lamp is also used for assessing lid tightness, judging centration and corneal coverage, assessing edge tightness and

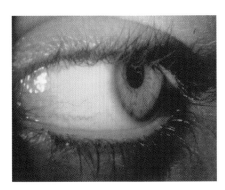

Figure 5.4
Lens lag.

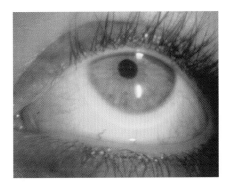

Figure 5.5
Lens sag.

viewing the lens tightness by using the push-up test.

Techniques

As with all contact lens fittings, an initial examination is required to judge patient suitability and evaluate patient needs. Chapter 1 covered this technique in depth.

Initial trial lens – choice and insertion

The first trial lens should be chosen using the basis of the following criteria:

Back vertex power – should be as close as possible to the patient's prescription to allow them to judge the benefits of contact lens wear correctly and to facilitate adaptation. If the exact power is not available, it is preferable that the lens is chosen to under-correct rather than to over-correct, to avoid accommodative spasms that could influence over-refraction. If monovision is to be tried (see Chapter 8), the lens should be chosen to be as close to the correct powers as possible.

Back optic zone radius – consulting the manufacturer's fitting guide should indicate which back optic zone radius (BOZR) to trial first for that particular lens design. In the majority of cases this should be done without regard to K-readings unless fitting patients with K-readings at the extreme range of normal.

Total diameter – must be larger than the HVID to allow for full corneal coverage in every position of gaze.

Lens thickness – some researchers have shown that, overall, lens bulk (thickness profile) is correlated to the initial comfort experienced by the patient,[4] although this finding has not been reported by others.[5]

Despite the apparent contraindication in the literature, it appears to make sense to fit a thinner lens to an apprehensive patient who is having an initial fitting to maximize the comfort response.

Adaptation period – fitting characteristics

Once the lenses have been inserted, the fit has to be assessed after a suitable settling period. Soft hydrogel lenses lose water as soon as they are placed on the eye, and this will change their parameters and, possibly, the fitting characteristics. Intuitively, it is important, therefore, that the fit is assessed once the lens is in equilibrium with the tear film. Classical soft hydrogel lens theory states that the lens should settle for 20–40 minutes before the fit is assessed. Brennan *et al*[6] looked at changes in fitting characteristics in low and high water content hydrogel lenses over an eight-hour wearing period. They found that lens movement decreased significantly over the first 25–30 minutes of wear. The most effective time to predict the final fitting characteristics was five minutes after the lens was inserted. It is proposed, therefore, that the fit should be assessed, initially, after five minutes and, if unacceptable at this time, another trial lens should be inserted.

Adaptation period – physiological and psychological characteristics

Five minutes is clearly insufficient for the practitioner to judge the physiological response to the lens and for the new patients to judge how they feel in lenses. A longer 'walkabout' trial allows the patient to appreciate what wearing contact lenses entails, although only gross physiological issues would be apparent. The longer the trial period is, then the better the practitioner's chances of judging the

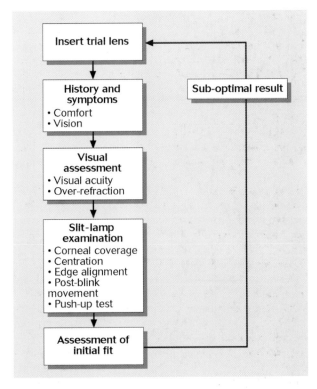

Figure 5.6
Schematic flow chart of soft contact lens fitting procedure.

physiological response to lenses, which will be particularly important in extended wear fitting. If a suitably long trial period can be managed, then practitioners should make the same assessments as they would during a routine aftercare examination.

Once the trial lens has been fitted, its assessment, as with all contact lenses, should be based on moving from the least to the most invasive technique.

Patient subjective response
Comfort – the patient should be aware of the

lens, but should also, generally, find it comfortable. There may be some initial discomfort after insertion due to differences between the osmolarity and pH of the lens storage solution and the patient's tears. This should, however, be quick to resolve. Lens sensation should be consistent, with no significant differences in lateral eye movement or blinking. As a general rule, initial comfort should be recorded as 7/10 or better.
Vision – with the appropriate over-refraction in place, vision should be stable and clear, although patients may notice

peripheral distortion and have initial difficulty in judging distances due to magnification changes. These should, however, soon resolve.

Over-refraction and visual acuity
A normal over-refraction should take place with binocular balancing. This balancing is required to overcome any accommodative spasm resulting from the foreign-body sensation of the lens in the eye. The refraction should have a clear endpoint and visual acuity should be stable and crisp. Variations in refraction or acuity could indicate a poor

Procedure	Ideal result	Variations from norm	Possible cause	Remedy
Comfort	Comfortable lens >7/10	Continual discomfort	Foreign body (FB) Thick lens Poor centration	Remove and replace lens Refit with thinner lens Tighten lens or change design
		Discomfort worse on blinking	Loose lens Edge stand-off	Tighten lens Change design
Vision	Crisp, clear, stable vision	Blurred vision Variable vision, after blinking	Incorrect power Loose lens	Over-refract Tighten lens
	Precise over-refraction	Variable over-refraction	Loose lens	Tighten lens
Centration	Full corneal coverage (1 mm to 2 mm overlap)	Greater than 2 mm conjunctival overlap Corneal exposure	Lens too large Too small lens Poor centration	Reduce total diameter Increase total diameter Tighten lens
	Centred in all positions of gaze	Corneal exposure at extremities of gaze	Loose lens Tight lids	Tighten lens Increase total diameter Try thinner lens
Edge alignment	Regular alignment to conjunctiva	Edge stand-off or fluting	Loose lens Peripheral lens design	Tighten lens Try different design
		Conjunctival indentation	Tight lens Peripheral lens design	Loosen lens Try different design
Primary gaze movement	0.2 mm to 0.4 mm movement	Less than 0.2 mm	Tight lens Hypotonic tears	Loosen lens, try different design Try different material
		More than 0.4 mm	Loose lens Excessive lacrimation See comfort	Tighten lens, try different design Check for FB Allow longer settling See comfort
Push-up test	Smooth recovery from push-up	Resistance to movement	Tight lens Hypotonic tears	Loosen lens Try different material
		Excessive movement and erratic recovery	Loose lens Excessive lacrimation See comfort	Tighten lens Check for FB Allow longer settling See comfort

Table 5.1
Key assessments made during the soft contact lens fitting procedure.

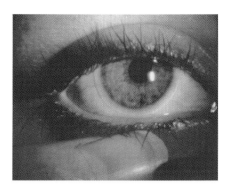

Figure 5.7(a)
(a) and (b) The push-up test.

lens fit, and the use of the retinoscope to collaborate this would be recommended.

Biomicroscope examination

Following over-refraction, the lens fit should be assessed at the slit-lamp. Diffuse direct illumination and medium to high magnification should be used to visualize the lens on the eye. The following assessments should be made:

Corneal coverage – with the eye in primary position, the lens should show full corneal coverage before, after and during the blink (Figure 5.1) and around 1 mm of conjunctival overlap.

Centration – the lens should be centred in the cornea in the primary position of gaze and should retain full corneal coverage of excursion gaze (lag), as shown in Figure 5.4, and upgaze (sag), as shown in Figure 5.5. Although tests and fitting guides recommend assessing both of these variables in judging the fit of a lens, studies indicate they have little predictive value in deciding if a lens is fitting successfully or not.

Primary gaze movement or post-blink movement – this should be judged or, ideally, measured using a graticule. This can be achieved by looking at the bottom of the lens during the blink or, if the lower lid obscures the inferior lens edge, at 4 or 8 o'clock. In some cases, it may be necessary to displace digitally the lower lid prior to making the assessment.

The ideal lens movement, as measured, should be 0.2 mm–0.4 mm. In modern, ultra thin, high water content and low elastic modulus lens materials and designs, the movement that is seen is often less than in older, thicker, lower water content designs. At times, it can be difficult for the practitioner to judge the fit on movement alone, and a better assessment of lens

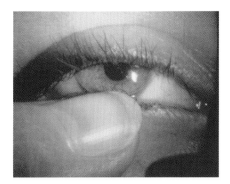

Figure 5.7(b)

dynamics can be made using the push-up test.

Push-up test – assessing the tightness of the lens is a measure of the fitting relationship of the lens with the eye. It is the most effective way of judging the dynamic fit. The operation of the test is shown in Figure 5.7. The practitioner moves the lens vertically, through pressure on the lower eyelid, using the finger. The lens is allowed to re-centre while being observed by the practitioner.

The practitioner assesses the relative ease with which the lens is displaced and the speed of its recovery to its original position. A percentage grade has been proposed, with 100 per cent representing a lens that is impossible to move and 0 per cent a lens that falls away from the cornea without lid support. An optimum fitting lens would be recorded as 50 per cent.[7]

The significance of the push-up test has been described by Martin *et al.*[8,9] Martin

showed that the movement of fluid beneath a soft lens is determined by the squeeze pressure, or the force between the front surface of the eye and the back surface of the lens. As squeeze pressure increases, the amount of fluid exchange decreases. Soft contact lens movement shows a poor correlation to squeeze pressure, which acts as a limiting factor, above which a lens shows no movement.

This correlation is illustrated in Figure 5.8, which is adapted from Martin *et al*, that shows that lenses may have a low enough squeeze pressure for fluid exchange to take place and yet show no movement. In comparison, tightness, as measured by the push-up test, showed a linear relationship with squeeze pressure (Figure 5.9), and so should be considered the arbitrator in judging lens fit.

Interpretation of findings

Consistent with good clinical practice in general, a particular observation should not be viewed in isolation. Interpreting results is facilitated by the practitioner following a structured routine, as shown in Figure 5.6.

Table 5.1 summarizes the key assessments made during the soft contact lens fitting procedure, and shows the characteristics of an ideal fit. The table also illustrates the sub-optimal responses that may be seen and suggests remedial actions. In this section, we will review the factors affecting fit and the remedial actions that may be taken.

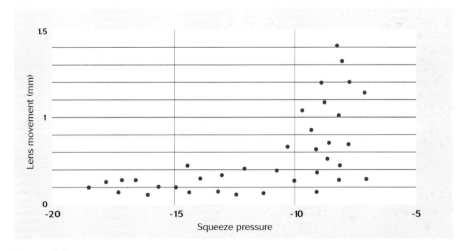

Figure 5.8
Relation between in vivo *lens movement and the squeeze pressure measured on the model eye (according to Martin* et al[8]*).*

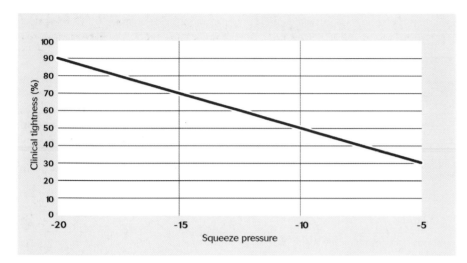

Figure 5.9
Relationship between the clinical assessment of lens fit and the measured squeeze pressure on the model eye (according to Martin et al)[8].

Ocular factors affecting lens fit

Ocular sag – this is a function of corneal shape factor, diameter and radius, as well as scleral radius and shape factor.[3] Without being able to assess accurately the variables affecting sag, an inspired approach of experimenting with trial lenses is the only way to judge the effect of the sag on the lens fit.

Corneal apex – a displaced corneal apex will lead to a decentred lens. Increasing the total diameter will expand the corneal coverage if it becomes exposed, while changes in the base curve will have little effect on centration in this case.

Lid pressure – tight lids often result in a high-riding lens and, possibly, excessive lens movement. Using a thin lens design and/or increasing lens diameter are management options. Loose lids generally have less effect on lens fits, although insufficient lens movement is a possible consequence.

Tear morphology – both pH and osmotic pressure can change lens parameters and affect the fit of the lens. A reduction in pH leads to a steepening of the ionic contact lens parameters, and one study[10] has shown that both ionic and non-ionic lenses steepen in fit as the tonicity of the tear film is reduced. This is clinically significant because if a satisfactory fit cannot be obtained with one contact lens material, then it might be worth changing the ionicity or water content to another material.

Lens variables affecting lens fit

Back optic zone radius – traditional soft contact lens fitting theory states that, as the BOZR increases, lenses move more and that,

as it decreases, lenses move less. Figure 5.10 shows this diagrammatically. Most practitioners have experienced situations in which the changing BOZR has a minimal, if any, effect on the lens fit, which has been supported by several studies. Numerous researchers[1,11] have shown that BOZR has no predictive value on lens movement.

Roseman's group also demonstrated that decreasing BOZR could improve centration without compromising the dynamic fit of the lens. This is not to say that changing the base curve will not affect movement, only that it may not have the predicted effect.

Total diameter – increasing the total diameter will expand the sag of the lens and tighten the fit, whereas reducing the total diameter will have the opposite effect. Total diameter might also be increased to improve corneal coverage in a lens fitted onto a cornea with a displaced apex.

Peripheral lens design – the peripheral design of a lens, which is the relationship between the front and back peripheral curves, has a marked effect on lens fit, as shown by Young et al.[5] As well as fitting characteristics, the peripheral design influences lens handling characteristics and comfort. The practitioner is, generally, unable to change these parameters, and, indeed, very little has been published that demonstrates the value of making changes. In practical terms, however, the practitioner should be aware that changing a lens from one design to another with the same BOZR and total diameter will not be a guarantee that the lens will fit in the same way. Table 5.2 suggests possible actions to change sub-optimal lens fitting characteristics.

Silicone hydrogels – The criteria described apply equally to silicone hydrogel lens fitting especially in relation to lens centration, corneal coverage and recovery following push-up test. However, current silicone hydrogel materials have a higher elastic modulus than soft hydrogel materials, resulting in approximately twice the lens stiffness. This may necessitate more than one fitting parameter to successfully fit a high percentage of the normal population. Careful observation of edge alignment of the lens to the bulbar conjunctiva should be made during biomicroscopic examination, as 'edge fluting' can be a significant reason for an unsuccessful fit.

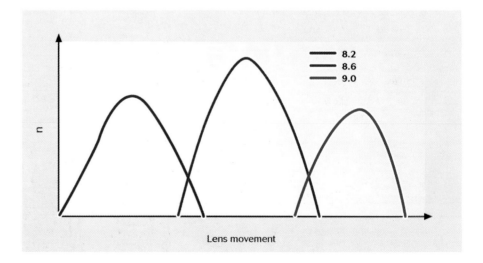

Figure 5.10a
The common falsely predicted effect of varying BOZR on lens movement.[1]

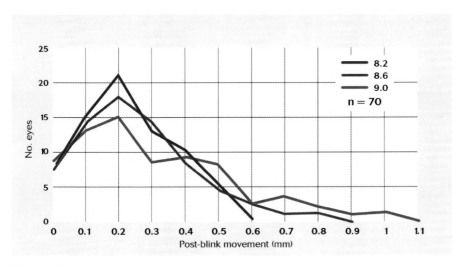

Figure 5.10b
The real effect of varying BOZR on soft lens post-blink movement (according to Young).[1]

Key points

- An ideally fitting soft contact lens should show the following attributes:

  Comfort (>8/10)

  Crisp, clear and stable vision

  Full corneal coverage in all gaze positions

  Regular edge alignment to the conjunctiva

  Post-blink movement of 0.2–0.4 mm

  Smooth recovery from push-up

- Lens fit and base curve selections are independent of K-readings

- The push-up test is of more value than post-blink movement

- Adopt a routine assessment, moving from the least to the most invasive technique

---

Summary

Although the practitioner has fewer parameters to choose from in deciding the optimal fit for a soft contact lens than with rigid lenses, it is still important that it is assessed accurately if the patient is to wear lenses successfully. This is perhaps even more critical while fitting silicone hydrogels, especially if prescribed on an extended wear basis. As soft lenses have become thinner, as hydrogel materials have been developed with lower elastic moduli and as lens designs have improved, the number of parameters required to fit a normal population has declined.

In many ways, contact lens texts have not always kept up with the understanding of the dynamics and the assessment of soft lens fitting.

This chapter has tried to provide a practical guide to the key aspects of modern soft contact lens fitting.

Of course, the process of soft contact lens fitting does not cease after the initial assessment. The effects of factors such as wearing time, environmental conditions and ocular physiology need to be monitored constantly. Ongoing aftercare is the key to continued contact lens success.

Question 5.1
Which of the following characteristics should a well fitting soft lens NOT show?
  A   Corneal coverage in all positions of gaze
  B   1 mm post blink movement
  C   Smooth return on push-up test
  D   Edge alignment to the conjunctiva
  E   High level of patient comfort and vision

Question 5.2
Central keratometry readings:
  A   Predict the BOZR to be chosen for a trial soft lens
  B   Provide baseline data of corneal contour
  C   Provide a means of judging tear quantity
  D   Correlate with the total sag of the best fitting soft lens
  E   Measure degree of peripheral corneal flattening

Question 5.3
When inserting a soft trial lens, symptoms of initial discomfort cannot be caused by:
  A   Differences between tear pH and the pH of the storage solutions
  B   Excessive lens movement caused by a loose lens and reflex tearing
  C   Differences between osmolarity of tears and storage solutions
  D   Insufficient lens movement
  E   Excessive edge stand-off from the conjunctiva

Question 5.4
The following assessments should NOT be made while viewing with the slit-lamp:
  A   Corneal centration
  B   Post-blink movement
  C   Visual stability
  D   Recovery following push-up test
  E   Conjunctival alignment

Question 5.5
Squeeze pressure:
  A   Is directly correlated with post-blink movement
  B   Is an assessment of the oxygen flux benefits
  C   Has a decreasing exponential relationship with lens tightness

Desired result	Action		
	First option	**Second option**	**Third option**
Loosen lens	Flatter BOZR	Reduce TD	Change material and/or design
Tighten lens	Steeper BOZR	Increase TD	Change material and/or design
Improve centration	Steeper BOZR	Increase TD	Change material and/or design

Table 5.2
Suggested actions to change soft lens fitting.

D Is a valuable means of assessing conjunctival alignment

E Has a linear relationship with lens tightness as measured by push-up test

Question 5.6
Which of the following external factors will not have an influence on lens fit?
A Corneal thickness
B Tear pH
C Corneal apex position
D Lid pressure
E Ocular sag

Question 5.7
Which of the following lens factors will not have an influence on lens fit?
A Peripheral lens design
B Water content of material
C Lens sagittal depth
D Lens total diameter
E Handling tint

Question 5.8
If a lens decentres, which of the following strategies could the practitioner use to improve the centration?
A Increase BOZR, maintain same TD
B Decrease BOZR, maintain same TD
C Increase BOZR, increase TD
D Increase lens thickness
E Decrease TD, maintain BOZR

Question 5.9
If a trial lens shows no significant post-blink movement, the practitioner should first:
A Use the push-up test to determine whether the fit is satisfactory
B Increase the BOZR
C Increase the water content of the lens
D Decrease the thickness of the lens
E Decrease the TD

Question 5.10
Which of the following will have the greatest impact on loosening a lens fit?
A Flatten BOZR, increase TD
B Steeper BOZR, reduce TD
C Flatten BOZR, reduce TD
D Steeper BOZR, increase TD
E Flatten BOZR only

References

1 Young, G. (1992) Soft lens fitting reassessed. *CL Spectrum* **7:12** 56–61.

2 Gundal, R., Cohen, H. and DiVergilio, D. (1986) Peripheral keratometry and soft lens fitting. *Int Eyecare* **2:12** 611–613.

3 Young, G. (1992) Ocular sagittal height and soft contact lens fit. *JBCLA* **15:1** 45–49.

4 Efron, N. (1986) Determinants of the initial comfort of hydrogel contact lenses. *Am J Optom Physiol Opt* **63:10** 819–823.

5 Young, G., Holden, B. and Cooke, G. (1993) Influence of soft contact lens design on clinical performance. *Optom Vis Sci* **70:5** 394–403.

6 Brennan, N. *et al.* (1994) Soft lens movement: temporal characteristics. *Optom Vis Sci* **71:6** 359–363.

7 Young, G. (1992) How to fit soft contact lenses. *JBCLA* **15:4** 179–180.

8 Martin, D. *et al.* (1989) A unifying parameter to describe the clinical mechanics of hydrogel contact lenses. *Optom Vis Sci* **66:2** 87–91.

9 Martin, D. and Holden, B. (1986) Forces developed beneath hydrogel contact lenses due to squeeze pressure. *Phys Med Biol* **30:** 635–649.

10 Little, S.A. and Bruce, A.S. (1995) Osmotic determinants of post-lens tear film morphology and hydrogel lens movement. *Ophthalmic Physiol Opt* **15:2** 117–124.

11 Roseman, M., Frost, A. and Lawley, M. (1993) Effects of base curve on the fit of thin, mid water contact lenses. *ICLC* **20:5 & 6** 95–101.

6
Rigid contact lens fitting

Introduction

Rigid gas-permeable (RGP) contact lens fitting is often regarded as a more complex procedure than soft lens fitting.

In reality, the number of decisions that have to be made by the practitioner are essentially the same when judging the fit of either lens. In addition, modern RGP lens designs can fit a wide range of the normal ametropic population, so practitioners need only specify the back optic zone radius (BOZR), total diameter (TD) and back vertex power (BVP) from a particular lens design for the manufacturer to produce the lens. While using custom-made multi-curve lens designs increases the practitioner flexibility in dealing with a range of corneal contours, many spherical and aspheric 'system' lens designs can cover most eventualities. Figure 6.1 summarizes basic contact lens parameters.

This chapter concentrates on basic procedures and techniques required to fit RGP lenses in routine contact lens practice with more specific detail on both multi-curve and aspheric designs available in the literature.[1]

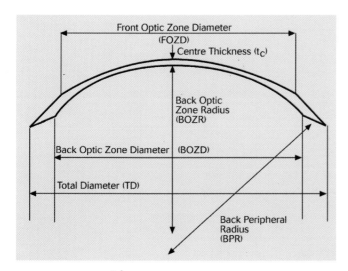

Figure 6.1
Diagrammatic representation of RGP lens dimensions.

The ideal RGP lens fit

As in soft contact lens fitting, the assessment of RGP lens fit involves the evaluation of both static and dynamic criteria. The ideal RGP fit should show the following characteristics.

Centration
The lens should remain centred over the pupil in primary gaze and maintain reasonable centration with each blink.

The goal of RGP lens centration is to ensure that the visual axis remains within the back optic zone diameter (BOZD) for as much time as possible to optimize visual acuity and avoid flare.

The lens should also remain on the cornea during all positions of gaze to minimize conjunctival staining from the periphery of the lens onto the limbal conjunctiva.

Corneal coverage
Unlike soft lenses, RGP lenses should be smaller than the corneal diameter. They should have a total diameter of at least 1.4 mm less than the horizontal visible iris diameter (HVID) to facilitate tear exchange under the lens and help optimize the alignment of the lens fit.

Dynamic fit
As well as allowing metabolic and tear debris to be removed from underneath the lens, the RGP lens must move to enable oxygen exchange due to the tear pump. Unlike soft lens fitting, there is a significant exchange of oxygen underneath an RGP lens during the blinking cycle.

Lens movement is one of the key characteristics of an ideal RGP fit. The lens should move around 1–1.5 mm with each blink. The movement should be smooth and unobstructed in the vertical plane, indicating a near alignment fit. Lens movement occurs either as a response to the eyelid force or by upper lid attachment. An immobile lens causes tears to stagnate beneath its surface, leading to corneal staining and distortion, while a lens with excessive movement causes patient discomfort, inconsistent vision and may also be associated with conjunctival staining.

Alignment
This is often the aspect of RGP lens fitting that receives most attention and, while important, should not be viewed in isolation of other aspects of lens fit. The ideal RGP fit should show alignment of the back surface of the lens with the cornea over most of the surface. A narrow band of edge clearance at the periphery is required to enable adequate tear exchange and to facilitate lens removal (Figure 6.2). The alignment of the back surface with the cornea allows the force of the lens to be distributed across the maximum bearing surface of the cornea. However, slight apical clearance and an area of light corneal touch in the mid-periphery will enhance lens centration; excessive touch can lead to tear stagnation, staining and/or distortion, while points of excessive clearance lead to an unstable lens fit in terms of centration, comfort and vision.

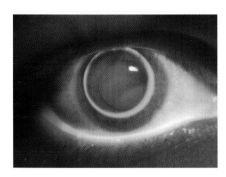

Figure 6.2
Fluorescein pattern of an ideal lens fit.

Patient response

When all the above are achieved, the patient should experience stable vision with the appropriate correction. The lens comfort should also be stable, depending on the degree of patient adaptation, but initial comfort will of course be less than that achieved with a soft lens.

Instrumentation

Keratometry

Lens selection

Central keratometry readings (K-readings) are the principal values used to select the initial trial, or empirically ordered, lens in RGP fitting. As well as assisting in choosing the appropriate BOZR, the K-reading in conjunction with the pupil size, may also be used to judge the appropriate BOZD. K-readings should be taken as the mean of three readings measured, which was described in Chapter 3. The assessment of peripheral K-readings is of limited value in routine contact lens practice, although in the absence of corneal topography it can be helpful in fitting the unusually contoured cornea, such as following refractive surgery or in cases of corneal pathology. The assessment of peripheral K-readings as a means of calculating the corneal shape factor can be of value in routine practice in interpreting unusual fluorescein patterns, which are seen in fitting both spherical and aspherical lens designs.

Baseline data

As in all contact lens practice, baseline K-readings must be recorded prior to fitting. An assessment of mire quality is especially valuable in RGP fitting as a rigid lens has the greatest capacity to cause distortion and alter this.

Tear quality

With the lens *in situ*, the keratometer can be used to record pre-lens tear break-up time.

Corneal astigmatism

The keratometer reading should be used together with the refraction result to determine the site and degree of any astigmatism. Spherical RGP lenses will only correct corneal astigmatism through neutralization by the tear lens. Of course, this cannot always be achieved with higher degrees of corneal astigmatism because of unstable fitting characteristics. In these cases, back surface toric RGP lenses are required to achieve a satisfactory fit.

If astigmatism is lenticular, a spherical RGP lens will have no effect on its correction. As a rule of thumb, 0.10 mm difference between K-readings equates to 0.50DC of corneal astigmatism. Table 6.1 shows some worked examples of this and some suggested suitable contact lens options, depending on the site of astigmatism.

Lens flexure

With the lens *in situ* on the eye, over K-readings will show any flexure of the lens on the eye. Flexure may occur either as the lens tries to assume the shape of a toric cornea under the influence of lid pressure, or as a lens becomes distorted with age or mishandling. Flexure is greatest with steep fitting lenses. If a satisfactory end-point of refraction cannot be obtained, then over K-readings can be used to confirm or eliminate flexure as a possible cause.

Corneal topography

Shape factor

The shape factor (or p value) of the cornea is the extent to which its shape varies from a sphere, which is the assumption made when K-readings are taken. Topography allows the practitioner to measure the shape factor of the cornea. This can be used to help choose the lens design and the extent to which the peripheral curves of the lens need flattening to maintain corneal alignment.

Some video keratoscopes have software that can recommend a lens design although, to date, the results from using such software during routine fitting have been unconvincing.[3]

Knowledge of the shape factor can be important in the analysis of some fluorescein patterns.

Ocular refraction			K-readings				Site of astigmatism	Contact lens options
Sphere	Cylinder	Axis	Flattest	Along	Steepest	Along		
-3.00	-2.00	180	8.00	180	7.60	90	Corneal	Spherical RGP, soft toric
-3.00	-2.00	180	8.00	180	8.00	90	Lenticular	FS toric RGP, soft toric
-3.00	0	0	8.00	180	7.60	90	Corneal	Spherical soft, toric RGP
-3.00	0	0	8.00	180	8.00	90	None	Spherical soft, spherical RGP
-3.00	-2.00	180	8.00	180	7.80	90	Mixed	FS toric RGP, soft toric
-3.00	-3.00	180	8.00	180	7.40	90	Corneal	Bi-toric RGP, soft toric

* FS = Front surface

Table 6.1
Examples to show how the site of astigmatism affects contact lens choice.

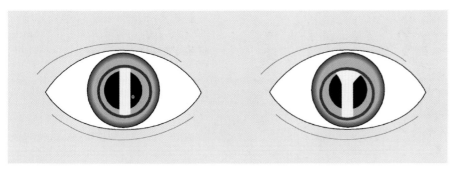

Figure 6.3
Retinoscopy reflex with centred RGP lens (left) and decentred lens (right).

Apex position and contour
Photokeratoscopy provides a contour map of the cornea, and this can be of value in looking for reasons to explain unusual fluorescein patterns or poorly centred lenses. Photokeratoscopy allows visualization of the apex of the cornea, which may not be in line with the visual axis, and hence shows the reason for a displaced lens. It will also show changes in contour due to pathology, surgery or even normal variations. As well as being a useful clinical aid, this technique assists the practitioner in explaining the mechanism of the lens fit to the patient.

Location of astigmatism
Corneal astigmatism can be calculated from any given two meridians from the centre to the periphery and can be displayed as a meridian contour map. The principal meridians and degree of astigmatism can be shown at various positions from the centre of the cornea. Importantly, this method of measurement demonstrates that corneal astigmatism is not necessarily uniform over the entire surface of the cornea, but varies according to the location on the cornea.

Retinoscopy

As well as playing a role in refraction, the retinoscope also allows the practitioner to judge pupil coverage by the BOZD of the lens. The retinoscopic reflex should be regular across the pupil. If the BOZD is not fully covering the pupil, then the reflex will become distorted at the transition between the central and peripheral radii (Figure 6.3).

Refraction
Over-refraction will provide the practitioner

with the necessary information to determine the correct BVP for an individual patient. Beyond this, it has two further important uses in RGP lens fitting.

Tear lens thickness
Optically, a RGP lens can be thought of as correcting ametropia in two ways: the replacing of the natural curvature of the cornea with a different curvature to correct the refractive error and the neutralization of the front surface of the cornea by the posterior lens surface. The power of this latter lens, the tear lens, can be calculated by over-refraction. This provides an invaluable means of assessing the lens/cornea alignment relationship.

Lens flexure
Over-refraction can also be used to judge lens flexure when an optimal visual result cannot be obtained with spherical lenses or over-refraction. If the practitioner is confident that the lens is correcting the corneal astigmatism and that there is no lenticular astigmatism present, then the flexure in the residual astigmatism produced is due to the lens flexing on the cornea.

PD ruler
The PD ruler (or preferably the graticule on the slit-lamp) should be used to measure the horizontal visible iris diameter (HVID), which may be used to choose the initial total diameter of the lens to trial. It should also be utilized to measure mean and maximum pupil diameters that will have an influence on the BOZD being selected. Finally, it would be used to measure vertical palpebral aperture size (VPA), both to assist in TD choice and as a baseline measurement as research has indicated that the VPA can decrease with RGP lens wear.

Biomicroscopy
Dynamic lens fit
Dynamic lens fit can be both assessed and measured using a slit-lamp with a graticule in the same way as soft lenses.

Lens/corneal alignment
- White light: an optic section can be used to judge the relationship of the lens to the cornea using white light and no fluorescein.
- Cobalt-blue light: the alignment of the back surface of the lens to the front surface of the eye is most effectively visualized using fluorescein. The fluorescein stains the tear film that makes up the tear lens. When the fluorescein is illuminated with the appropriate wavelength of blue light it fluoresces a green colour. The intensity of the green colour is a function of the thickness of the fluorescein film. The thicker the film, the more yellow the appearance.[4]

Fluorescein in the tears fills the space between the back surface of the lens and the anterior corneal surface. When excited with the cobalt-blue filter, the distance between the two surfaces is represented by the intensity of the fluorescent light, with the brighter the colour seen, the greater the gap and vice versa. By looking at the change in intensity of the fluorescein across the lens, the distance between the posterior lens surface and the anterior corneal surface can be visualized, the so-called fluorescein pattern (Figure 6.2).

As in the use of fluorescein for other purposes, the use of a yellow barrier filter over the slit-lamp eyepiece will assist in increasing the contrast between the yellow fluorescein and the background. In carrying out this technique, it is important to ensure that excessive fluorescein is not placed in the eye, as this will make the interpretation of the fit more difficult.

Burton lamp
Fluorescein fit
The Burton lamp is an ultraviolet light source mounted with a magnifying glass in a rectangular frame. It allows the practitioner to view fluorescein patterns using the UV light to excite the fluorescein.

The disadvantages are that the magnification is not as good as that achieved with the slit-lamp and is ineffective when used with lenses that have a UV inhibitor in the polymer. For this type of lens, the cobalt-blue light on the slit-lamp is the preferred option.

Astigmatism (by keratometer)	Approximate BOZR
Spherical - 0.75D	Fit on flattest keratometer reading
0.50 – 1.00D	Fit on flattest keratometry reading to 0.05 steeper than the flattest keratometer reading
1.00 – 2.50D	Fit near flattest keratometer reading (0.05 to 0.10 steeper at most) to minimize flexure and achive good acuity with a spherical lens[5]
Over 2.50D	A toroidal back optic zone is recommended

Table 6.2
Choice of BOZR based on K-readings for spherical RGP lenses (BOZD = 7.50).

Pupil size
Maximum pupil size can be measured in a darkened room with the eye illuminated using the UV light on the Burton lamp. The pupil can then be easily visualized against the fluorescence of the crystalline lens.

Techniques

As with all contact lens fittings, an initial examination is required to judge patient suitability and evaluate patient needs.

Initial trial lens - choice and insertion

With the recent concerns from the Department of Health regarding the theoretical possibility of the transfer of variant CJD via the use of reusable contact lenses, the use of fitting/trial sets for routine RGP fitting has become less common apart from when fitting more complex designs.

At this time, fitting usually requires the practitioner to order a contact lens empirically based upon initial measurements and the fit and power may then be adjusted if necessary. It is this initial lens that is referred to as the trial lens throughout the rest of this chapter and should be chosen using the following criteria:

Back vertex power

Where possible, this should be as close as possible to the patient's final prescription, both to provide the patient with as natural vision as possible and to minimize the potential changes in fit from variation in power. As the centre of gravity and edge design of a plus-powered lens is in a different position to a minus lens, the fit may be different. It is important, therefore, that hypermetropes

be assessed with positively powered lenses and vice versa.

If there is a choice of prescription, the practitioner should err towards under-correction rather than over-correction of myopes to minimize the chances of accommodative spasm.

Back optic zone radius

The design of RGP lenses may be spherical, aspherical or a combination of both. Spherical lenses may be bi-curve, tri-curve or multi-curve and with each different BOZR the peripheral curve design can result in a constant axial edge lift or constant axial edge clearance design. Generally, aspheric designs vary from those with a fixed elliptical curve (e.g. e = 0.5) to those where the eccentricity of the curve varies from the centre of the lens to the edge (e.g. polynomial or variable eccentricity).

- Spherical lenses: the initial trial lens should be chosen, based on the K-readings, using either the manufacturer's recommendations for a particular lens design or the values shown in Table 6.2. The practitioner should note that the values provided for the initial trial lens fitting are guidelines only.
- Aspherical lenses: elliptical aspheric lenses generally need a flatter fitting than spherical lenses to provide alignment across the corneal surface, however polynomial and variable eccentricity aspheric designs can be fitted in very much the same way as spherical designs. The initial trial lens should be fitted in accordance with the manufacturer's recommendation which is generally on, or slightly flatter, than the flattest K.

Total diameter

The total diameter (TD) chosen is based upon the HVID and lid position. As a generalization, the TD should be at least 1.4 mm smaller than the HVID. The smaller the palpebral aperture, the smaller the TD should be. Guillon recommends that the choice is made in accordance with Figure 6.4.

Once again, the initial trial lens recommendation is a guide from which the optimal lens fit may be judged.

Centre thickness

For physiological reasons, the lenses should be made as thin as possible to maximize oxygen transmissibility. For most materials

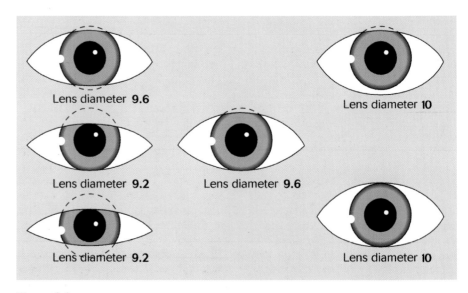

Figure 6.4
Selection of rigid lens total diameter as a function of eyelid position, according to Guillon.[6]

	+2	+1	0	-1	-2
Central fit	Excessively steep	Slightly steep	Alignment	Slightly flat	Excessively flat
Peripheral fit Width	Extremely wide (0.4 mm)	Slightly wide (0.3 to 0.4 mm)	Optimal (0.2 to 0.3 mm)	Slightly narrow (0.1 to 0.2 mm)	Extremely narrow (<0.1 mm)
Height	Excessive	More than optimal	Optimal	Less than optimal	Insufficient
Mid-peripheral fit	Hard well-defined contact	Poorly defined contact	No contact		

Table 6.3
Grading of fluorescein fit, adapted from Guillon.[6]

today, the realistic minimal centre thickness is approximately 0.14 mm.

Back optic zone diameter

With 'system' lenses, the practitioner often has little control over this parameter, although it should be considered in relation to pupil size. The BOZD should be at least 1 mm larger than average pupil size in normal room illumination to avoid flare. The BOZD also has most influence on the corneal alignment of any of the posterior diameters. As the corneal K-readings flatten, a larger BOZD should be considered to maintain alignment over the cornea.

Material

It could be argued that the lens material used for the lens fitting assessment should ideally be the same as the intended material for the final lens prescribed. This is to minimize the possibility of the prescription lens behaving differently from the initial lens assessed in terms of flexure, centration or wetting.

For physiological reasons, materials of Dk >50 should be routinely considered for daily wear of RGP lenses. Rigid gas-permeable materials used today include silicone acrylates and fluorosilicone acrylate, the latter having the advantage of better wettability and fewer deposits but require more careful manufacture and can be brittle if too thin.

Insertion and adaptation

Insertion

New lenses should be hydrated in a soaking solution for at least 24 hours before an accurate assessment of the fit can be made. Immediately prior to insertion, patients should be instructed on the foreign-body sensation they are likely to experience with the lens *in situ*. They should also be asked to look downwards once the lens is inserted. This minimizes the action of the lid on the lens edge and reduces the foreign-body sensation.

Once the lens has been inserted, lifting the upper eyelid will enable the practitioner to judge whether or not any discomfort is due to normal adaptation (in which case it will disappear when the lid is lifted) or a foreign body trapped between the lids (in which case it will remain).

Adaptation

Once reflex tearing has stopped, the fit of the lens can be grossly assessed, normally after approximately five minutes. At this stage, the assessment is only to ensure that the lens is stable enough for a reasonable trial period. Assessments should be made with white light and the naked eye to check overall lens centration and then a gross fluorescein fit assessment. If a reasonable fit is obtained, patients should be sent for a longer trial period to enable them to judge their subjective response and allow some degree of adaptation. This period should be a minimum of 30 minutes.

Subjective response

At the end of the tolerance period, the patient should be tolerably aware of the lenses and reflex lacrimation should have subsided. If the lens is near the correct power, the patient should report stable vision in all positions of gaze.

Assessment of fit

Fit assessment should be made, starting with the least invasive technique and moving on to the most invasive to minimize the stimulation of reflex tearing, which could alter the fit.

Over-refraction and visual acuity

A spherical over-refraction should be conducted initially with binocular balancing to relax the accommodation that may have been induced from the foreign-body sensation of the lens *in situ*. The visual acuity should be crisp and stable with a precise end-point of refraction. If unstable or unacceptable acuity is found, a cylindrical refraction should be carried out. The refraction should be both subjective and objective using the retinoscope. The finding should be recorded so that tear lens power can be calculated and adjustments made to the central fit if necessary.

White light

Under white light and with the naked eye, the practitioner should judge the centration of the lens in primary gaze and on lateral eye movement. In addition to centration, the movement with blink should be judged, the lens should move with each blink under the influence of the upper eyelid and return to cover the pupil immediately afterwards.

Fluorescein assessment

With the patient at the slit-lamp or using the Burton lamp, a fluorescein assessment of the fit should be carried out. A minimal amount of fluorescein should be inserted into the conjunctival sac and the patient should be asked to blink. The practitioner should then systematically assess the brightness of the fluorescein in three regions: central, mid-peripheral and peripheral. A simple grading scale has been advocated by Guillon to assess the lens fit (Table 6.3).

Put simply, if fluorescein is seen under the lens during assessment then it can range from a little (alignment or slight apical clearance) to a moderate amount (+1) or an excessive amount (+2). If it is

Symptom	Possible causes	Remedy
Poor comfort	Excess movement	Tighten fit
	Excess edge clearance	Reduce edge clearance
	Edge too thick	Thinner edge
	Foreign body	Remove and replace lens
	Damaged lens edge	Replace lens
	Astigmatic cornea	Modify fit
		Consider an aspheric design
		Consider a toric design
	Patient sensitivity	Thinner lens design
		Increase total diameter
		Soft lens
	Poor wetting	Remove and clean lens
		Change material
Poor vision	Refractive shape	Refract and change power
	Corneal shape change	Assess fit and modify
	Residual astigmatism	Toric lens
	Flexure	Flatten fit
		Change material
	Deposits	Clean lens
	Heavy surface scratches	Polish or replace lens
	Poor wetting	Remove and clean lens
		Replace lens if old
		Change material

Table 6.4
Possible causes of patient symptoms with RGP lenses.

difficult to judge because of an apparent even film of fluorescein this is an alignment fit. It is generally easier to detect a steep fit than a flat fit. This may be worth bearing in mind when selecting the first trial lens.

Interpretation of findings

Subjective response
Comfort with RGP lenses is initially less than with soft lenses although, following a 30-minute adaptation period, the patient should report no more than lens sensation. If 'pain' is reported, together with excessive reflex tearing, then the lens needs modification. Reasons for poor comfort and the remedial actions are summarized in Table 6.4.

Vision and visual acuity should be stable and crisp, with the correct spherical over-correction in place. If a stable result cannot be obtained with spherical lenses, a cylindrical over-correction should be attempted. A stable result indicates that residual astigmatism exists within the optical correction and that a toric lens may be required.

Before going ahead with a toric fit, the practitioner should analyse the results of the over-correction to identify the site of the residual astigmatism and make sure that it is not lens flexure that is causing the poor vision.

If no site for the astigmatism can be found, or it is variable, the most likely cause is lens flexure. In cases of lens flexure, changes to the lens/eye fitting relationship are the preferred management option.

Table 6.4 summarizes the causes of poor vision and the management options.

Over-refraction
Determining the over-refraction allows the tear lens to be calculated. It is the difference in power between the refraction at the corneal plane and the power of the contact lens needed to correct the ametropia. The power of the tear lens is an invaluable means of assessing the alignment of the lens to the cornea. If the lens is fitting steeply, a positive tear lens will result and the power of the contact lens will require less plus or more minus than the ocular refraction. If the lens is fitting flatter than the cornea, the tear lens will be negative and the converse will apply (Figure 6.5).

Table 6.5 shows some worked examples of different tear lenses. A general guide towards calculating tear lens powers is that 0.50DS difference in over-refraction relates to 0.10 mm difference between lens radius and corneal radius.

Lens centration
The lens should remain centred over the visual axis between blinks and on lateral gaze. Some higher minus-powered lenses 'hook' on to the upper eyelid, which holds the lens in position. In these cases, the lens moves with the lid.

The same effect can be obtained by ordering a lens with a front surface negative peripheral carrier, which may be of value in fitting hypermetropes whose lenses continually drop. As long as the BOZD covers the pupil and the edge does not cause

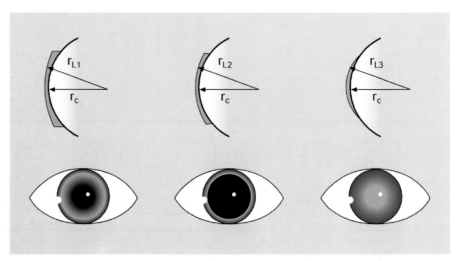

Figure 6.5
Tear lens thickness.

Ocular refraction	CL power in air	Over-refraction	Tear lens	Fitting relationship
−3.00	−3.00	0	0	Alignment
−3.00	−2.50	0	−0.50	Flat
−3.00	−3.50	0	+0.50	Steep
−3.00	−3.00	−0.50	+0.50	Steep
−3.00	−3.00	+0.50	−0.50	Flat

Table 6.5
Examples to show how the tear lens power can be used to assess the lens/cornea alignment.

excessive pressure on the limbal region, some degree of decentration is acceptable on rigid contact lens fitting. If either of these result in fluctuation of vision, glare/haloes, conjunctival or limbal staining, the lens fit needs modifying. Table 6.6 shows options available to improve the centration of a decentred lens.

Lens movement
The lens should show sufficient vertical movement to allow tear exchange to take place. Typically, this is around 1 mm to 1.5 mm. Excessive movement leads to poor comfort, vision and the potential for conjunctival staining. Insufficient movement leads to tear stagnation, corneal staining

and distortion. Options to increase or decrease lens movements are given in Table 6.7.

Fluorescein patterns
Figure 6.6 shows a series of fluorescein patterns, with grading and recommended management options. Interpretation of fluorescein patterns should not be undertaken in isolation; confirmation of the lens/eye relationship should be made by calculating the tear lens and a steep looking fit should show a positive tear lens and vice versa.

Occasionally, a steep or flat-looking fit may occur, even when the BOZR of the lens and the K-readings of the cornea appear to

match one another exactly. There are two reasons for this: the trial lens has the incorrect BOZR or it is due to the corneal shape factor. If the cornea has a lower than average p value (i.e. p less than 0.75), it flattens out at a faster than normal rate towards the periphery and consequently, a spherical lens of the same central radius may show central pooling (Figure 6.7). The fit will have to be modified in the same way as dealing with a steep-fitting lens.

Interdependency of fitting variables
Every variable in RGP lens design has an interdependency on other variables. If there is a need to change one parameter on the lens, such as BOZD, then, if the same

---

Key points

- An ideally fitting rigid contact lens should show the following attributes:
  Comfort (>7/10) once adapted
  Adequate centration (no limbal overlap, BOZD centred over pupil)
  TD approx 1.4 mm smaller than the HVID 1–1.5 mm smooth movement with each blink
  Lens alignment over most of the corneal surface, or alignment along the flatter meridian in the case of toric corneas
  Narrow band of edge clearance.
- Tear lens power should be calculated to confirm an alignment fit.
- The use of a slit-lamp to view the fluorescein fit provides a better overall assessment than a Burton lamp.
- Adapt a routine assessment, moving from the least to the most invasive technique.

Lens position	Possible causes	Remedy
Continually high, not dropping after blink	Flat peripheral zone Widen peripheral zone Too large TD Lens too thick With-the-rule cyl	Steepen periphery Narrow periphery Reduce TD Reduce Tc and/or Te BS toric design Toric periphery design
Continually low/rapid drop after blink	Lens too small Lens too thick No lid attachment	Increase TD Reduce Tc Add peripheral negative carrier
Continually to one side	Displaced corneal apex Lens too small Lens too flat Against-the-rule cyl	Increase TD Soft lens Increase TD Steepen design BS toric design Toric periphery design
Stationary Excessive decentration beyond limbus	Lens too steep Excess lacrimation Lens too flat Excess corneal cyl	Flatten fit See symptoms Steepen design BS toric design

*BS = Back surface

Table 6.6
Management of lens decentration.

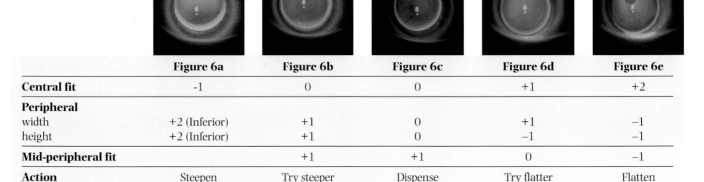

	Figure 6a	Figure 6b	Figure 6c	Figure 6d	Figure 6e
Central fit	-1	0	0	+1	+2
Peripheral					
width	+2 (Inferior)	+1	0	+1	-1
height	+2 (Inferior)	+1	0	-1	-1
Mid-peripheral fit		+1	+1	0	-1
Action	Steepen BOZR	Try steeper BOZR	Dispense	Try flatter BOZR	Flatten BOZR

Figure 6.6
Interpretation of fluorescein patterns (Courtesy of David Ruston).

fitting relationship is to be maintained, the BOZR also has to be altered to maintain the same sagittal height. Changing either the BOZD or the BOZR will also alter the tear lens and hence the power of the lens/eye system. The extent of these changes will depend upon, to some extent, the ocular parameters and the lens material characteristics. Table 6.8 summarizes the basic rules of thumb in making alterations to lens parameters.

Summary

The practitioner has many parameters to choose from in deciding the optimal fit for a rigid lens. Although system-designed lenses are suitable for many, optimum comfort or visual acuity should not be compromised if

an ideal fit cannot be achieved. Skilled laboratories can design lenses to exact specifications, if required. As with all contact lens practice, a systematic approach should be utilized. Changes to lens parameters should not be made unless there is a logical reason to do so.

Question 6.1
A well fitting RGP lens should ideally show:
- A Full corneal coverage in all positions of gaze
- B No vertical post-blink movement
- C Pupil coverage by the BOZD
- D Central apical corneal contact
- E No edge clearance

Question 6.2
A difference of 0.4 mm between steepest

and flattest keratometry readings equates approximately to:
- A 4.00D of corneal astigmatism
- B 1.00D of lenticular astigmatism
- C 2.00D of corneal astigmatism
- D 1.00D of corneal astigmatism
- E 2.00D of lenticular astigmatism

Question 6.3
In which of the following prescriptions will a spherical RGP lens not provide satisfactory vision?
- A Rx: -2.00 DS
  K: 7.60 al 180 - 7.60 al 90
- B Rx: -2.00 DS/-2.00DC × 180
  K: 7.60 al 180 - 7.20 al 90
- C Rx: -2.00 DS/-2.00DC × 180
  K: 7.60 al 180 - 7.50 al 90
- D Rx: -5.00/+2.00 × 180
  K: 8.00 al 90 - 7.60 al 180
- E Rx: −3.00/−2.00 × 90
  K: 7.60 al 180 - 8.00 al 90

Question 6.4
Which of the following will over-refraction not give information about:
- A Alignment of back surface of lens to cornea
- B Flexure of lens
- C Required lens power
- D Degree of corneal eccentricity
- E Tear lens thickness

Question 6.5
A patient has K-readings of 7.80 al 180 and 7.40 al 90. Which spherical back surface lens should be the trial lens of first choice?

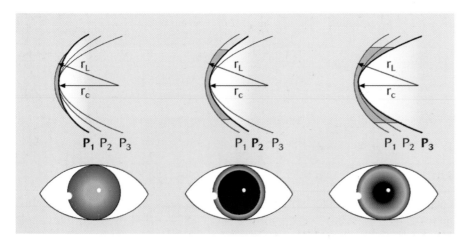

Figure 6.7
Effect of corneal shape factor on fluorescein fit.

Strategy	Variable			
	BOZR	**BOZD**	**TD**	**Tc**
Increase movement	Increase	Decrease	Decrease	Increase
Decrease movement	Decrease	Increase	Increase	Decrease

Table 6.7
Management of lens movement.

A 7.40
B 7.20
C 7.90
D 7.70
E 7.60

Question 6.6
A patient complains of poor comfort while wearing an RGP lens. This is unlikely to be caused by:
A Excess lens movement
B Trapped foreign body
C Excess edge clearance
D Lenticular astigmatism
E Poor wetting

Question 6.7
Which of the following is unlikely to be a cause of poor vision in an RGP lens wearer?
A Lens flexure
B Excess edge clearance
C Poor wetting
D Residual astigmatism
E Change in corneal shape

Question 6.8
A patient experiences 'flare' resulting from an RGP lens that rides high and does not drop with the blink. Which of the following statements is true?
A The patient probably has against the rule astigmatism
B The lens probably needs a larger TD and BOZD
C The patient may require a toric front surface design
D The lens probably requires cleaning and polishing
E The lens material probably needs changing

Question 6.9
Which of the following would not cause decentration of an RGP lens?
A Displaced corneal apex
B Against the rule astigmatism

C Excessive lacrimation
D Total diameter too small
E Total diameter too large

Question 6.10
Which of the following lenses should be chosen to achieve the same optical corrections as a lens with a BOZR of 7.80 and a power of +3.00?
A 7.90 + 3.50
B 7.90 + 2.50
C 7.90 + 3.25
D 7.90 + 2.75
E 7.85 + 3.25

References

1 Atkinson, T.C.O. (1985) A computer assisted and clinical assessment of current trends in gas permeable lens design. *Optician* **189:4976** 16–22.
2 Meyler, J.G. and Ruston, D.M. (1994) Rigid gas permeable aspheric back surface contact lenses – a review. *Optician* **208:5467** 22–30.
3 Szczotka, L., Capretta, D.M. and Lass, J.H. (1994) Clinical evaluation of a computerized topography software method for fitting rigid gas-permeable contact lenses. *CLAO Journal* **20:4** 231–236.
4 Cooke, G. and Young, G. (1986) The use of computer-simulated fluorescein patterns in rigid lens design. *Trans BCLA* 21–26.
5 Stone, J. and Collins, C. (1984) Flexure of gas permeable lenses on toroidal corneas. *Optician* **188:4951** 8–10.

Further reading

Guillon, M. (1994) Basic contact lens fitting. In: Rub, M., Guillon, M. (eds). *Contact Lens Practice*. Chapman and Hall Medical, 587–622.
Phillips, A.J. (1997) Rigid gas-permeable

A change of BOZR of 0.05 mm is equivalent to 0.25D change in power if radius is in region 7.80 mm
A change of BOZD of 0.05 mm requires the BOZR be changed by 0.05 mm to maintain the same fluorescein pattern

Table 6.8
Basic rules of thumb.

and corneal lens fitting. In: Phillips, A.J. and Speedwell, L. (eds). *Contact Lenses* 4th edn. Butterworth-Heinemann, 313–357.
Gasson, A. and Morris, J. (1998) *The Contact Lens Manual*. Butterworth-Heinemann.

7
Soft toric contact lens fitting

Introduction

Soft toric contact lens fitting used to be regarded as a 'speciality', which was only to be undertaken by experienced practitioners following extensive training and experience. In recent years, however, the number of designs available to the practitioner has increased and the fitting approach simplified.

Soft torics have moved away from being custom-made individual products requiring large fitting sets and long delivery times.

Soft torics are now available from stock and with an ever-increasing number offering the benefits of disposability; toric lenses can be fitted empirically or from comprehensive in-practice fitting banks. The latter now makes trialling astigmatic patients with single-use toric disposable lenses as convenient as spherical lens fitting. One of the reasons for this increase in the simplicity of fitting toric lenses has been advances in manufacturing technology. The advent of new low-cost moulding technology and wet moulding techniques allowing the lens to remain hydrated throughout manufacture, has led to improvements in contact lens reproducibility and optical quality. This should give practitioners greater confidence that the lens being dispensed is the same as the lens being ordered.

As well as improving the simplicity of the fitting and lens quality, manufacturers have also been able to further enhance the design of toric lenses, creating lenses that are thinner, more comfortable and show more consistent stabilization than many of the early designs. As manufacturing reliability has increased, so has the availability of soft toric lenses, in terms of the materials from which they are made. Torics are now available in thinner designs or higher water content polymers, improving the physiological performance of the lens on the eye.

So should soft torics be regarded as an integral, routine part of contact lens practice? We believe the answer is yes.

Around 16 per cent of prescriptions have more than 1.00DC of astigmatism (Table 7.1) which increases to over 30 per cent of the ametropic population with 0.75D or more of refactive astigmatism.[1] To correct this refractive error, the practitioner has a number of alternative choices:

Spherical RGP lenses

Rigid gas-permeable lens will correct corneal astigmatism, however, a spherical RGP lens will not correct lenticular astigmatism. In cases of high corneal toricity the fit might become unstable and a toric periphery or full toric back surface will be required. The advantage of a spherical RGP lens to correct astigmatism is the relative ease of the fit, while the disadvantages are the reduced comfort associated with rigid lenses, the difficulty in obtaining a well-centred lens in some cases (Figure 7.1 (a)) and the frequent problem of 3 and 9 o'clock staining.

Toric periphery or full-toric RGP lenses

Introducing a toroidal surface to the back of the lens will improve its physical fit on the cornea. A toric periphery has the advantage of being independent of the visual component of the correction, although it might be inadequate in achieving full stability of fit.

One recently described disadvantage of a toric periphery is that in the manufacture of some lenses it is often impossible to duplicate the actual parameters.[2] This leads to variation in the actual lens parameters that might make reordering an identical lens impossible.

Having a full toric back surface on the lens provides the best option in achieving an alignment fit (Figure 7.1 (b)). A full toric

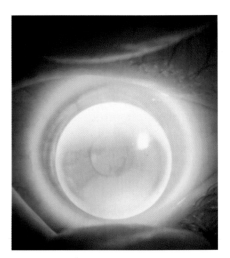

Figure 7.1 Different lens designs on a cornea with 3.00 DC of astigmatism
(a) C3 spherical RGP lens (courtesy of Eric Papas).

Power of correction cylinder (D)	Percentage of total sample (%)	Percentage of astigmatic lenses (%)
0	32.0	
0.25–0.50	34.6	50.9
0.75–1.00	17.7	26.0
1.25–2.00	9.8	14.4
2.25–3.00	3.8	5.6
3.25–4.00	1.5	2.2
Over 4.00	0.6	0.9

Table7.1
Incidence of astigmatism, from Bennett.[1]

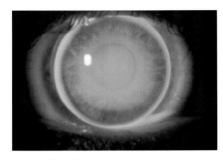

Figure 7.1(b)
Back-surface toric RGP lens (courtesy of Eric Papas).

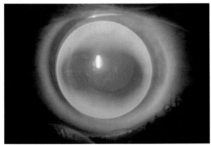

Figure 7.1(c)
Elliptical RGP lens design (courtesy of Eric Papas).

back surface will, however, require the practitioner, or the laboratory, to calculate the powers needed on the front surface to neutralize any induced astigmatism and fully correct the patient's ametropia.

A toric lens on a toric cornea should be a more comfortable option than a spherical lens on a toric eye, although the usual problem of rigid lens adaptation still needs to be addressed. Further information on fitting rigid toric lenses can be obtained from various publications.[3,4]

Elliptical RGP lens
Elliptical RGP lenses have been reported as correcting up to 1.00DC more corneal astigmatism than a spherical design[5], although such designs have only a marginal benefit when improving the fitting relationship along the steeper meridian of more toric corneas (>2.50D).

As with spherical lenses, they need to be fitted on, or flatter than, the flattest K-reading to avoid the lens flexing on the eye (Figure 7.1 (c)). The stability of the lens fit will be the limiting factor in the degree of astigmatism for which this lens design will be suitable.

Thick soft lenses
An often-quoted strategy for correcting astigmatism with soft lenses is to increase

the thickness of the lens. The theory behind this is that a thicker lens will drape less on the cornea and so mask more astigmatism.

The best controlled study carried out to investigate this detected no significant difference in vision between two soft lenses that were identical, apart from in thickness.[6]

The study did, however, show that for some individual patients, vision was improved with the thicker lenses. This suggests that increasing the thickness might have some optical benefit for a limited number of individuals. The disadvantage of this technique is that as the thickness increases, the oxygen supply decreases and the physiological compromise is much greater.

Aspheric hydrogel surfaces
The use of aspheric front surfaces to correct the spherical aberration in the lens/eye system has been shown to produce better visual performance due to a reduction in size of the total blur circle even though the eye remains astigmatic. Their use in correcting astigmatism is poorly documented although some work has been published showing that aspheric designs might provide as good visual acuity as a soft toric lens for up to 1.50DC of astigmatism.[7] However, one would expect that visual performance would depend upon the interaction of the optical characteristics of the particular lens design with the aberrations of the eyes of the wearer. Consequently, variations in ocular aberration between individuals may explain in part why lenses of this type meet the needs of some wearers but not others.

Soft toric lens
The final option for the practitioner is to fit a soft toric lens. This has the comfort advantage of soft material and generally improved visual performance over the other soft lens options discussed. The rest of this chapter will discuss soft toric contact lens fitting in practice.

Instrumentation

The basic instrumentation required for soft toric lens fitting is the same as that needed to fit regular soft lenses. A slit-lamp having a graticule with a protractor is of particular value in soft toric lens fitting to assist in locating the axis. If this is not available,

rotation of the slit beam and a scale indicating the degree of rotation can be helpful.

Lens trial

The ideal system would be to have a comprehensive bank of single-use trial lenses in practice to allow astigmatic patients to experience lens wear as conveniently as their spherical counterparts. With the recent advice surrounding new variant CJD, the alternative option is empirical fitting, whether fitting a disposable lens or conventional stock toric lens. Regardless of the approach taken, a lens must be assessed on the eye to allow the practitioner to assess both the physical fit of the lens and its rotational behaviour, which will determine the optical result. Maintaining the rotational stability of the lens is the key to successful soft toric fitting.

Surface toricity
A rigid toric lens maintains its position on the cornea through the alignment of the back surface of the lens with the toric cornea assuming that the cornea has sufficient toricity to justify the toric fitting. If a soft lens is produced with a toric back surface, its reduced modulus of elasticity means the lens will still drape and so rotate on the eye. For this reason, toric back surface lenses are equally suitable to fit on spherical corneas when correcting lenticular astigmatism helped further by the spherical fitting curve which surrounds the back surface toric optic portion present in more recent designs. However, to keep the astigmatic correction of the lens in align-

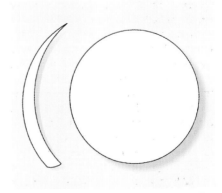

Figure 7.2(a)
Cross-section through a prism-ballasted soft toric lens, showing the variation in thickness.

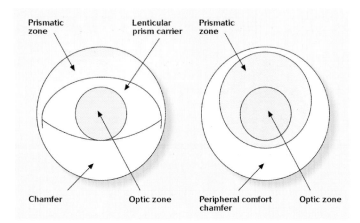

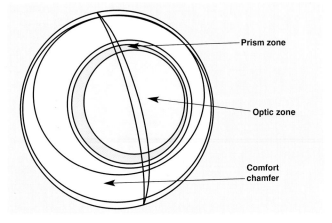

Figure 7.2 (b)
A prism-stabilized soft toric lens, showing the prism free central optic zone, and the peripheral carrier with prism and comfort chamfer, from Grant.[9]

Figure 7.2 (c)
A prism-stabilized soft toric lens, showing the prism free central optic zone, and the peripheral carrier with prism and comfort chamfer to allow control of lens thickness with different lens powers (adapted from Cox et al.)[12].

ment to that of the eye, the lens must be held in position. There are two basic ways to achieve this:
• Prism stabilization
• Dynamic stabilization

Truncating the lens by removing part of the lower portion of the prism is generally no longer carried out (Figure 7.3).

Prism stabilization
This was the first and, although considerably adapted over the years, is still the most common means of stabilizing a lens in the eye. In principle (Figure 7.2 (a)), the lens is produced with an increasingly thicker profile towards its base. The thinner portion of the lens locates under the upper eyelid, which then squeezes the thicker portion of the lens towards the lower lid (the so-called watermelon seed principle). Gravity has been shown not to play a part in the axis location.[8]

The increase in the thickness of the lens naturally means that less oxygen is transmitted through the material and can

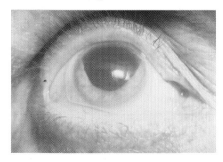

Figure 7.3
Truncated soft toric lens.

also lead to a decrease in comfort, especially against the lower lid. To overcome this, manufacturers remove as much of the prism as possible from the lens through 360 degree comfort chamfers and eccentric lenticulation, which are designed to reduce the thickness of the lens,[9] (Figure 7.2 (b)). In addition, prism stabilized lens designs have seen further refinements resulting in prism-free optics and prism that is restricted to the lens periphery.[10,11]

Other designs aim to control the thickness profile vertically to limit unwanted rotational forces and minimize differences in stabilization between lenses of different power and cylinder axis[12] (Figure 7.2(c)).

Dynamic stabilization
Dynamic stabilized lenses also rely on the interaction between lids and the lens to achieve stabilization. Both eyelids play an active role unlike with prism-stabilized designs that involve interaction primarily from the upper lid.

Stabilization is achieved by either designing a thin zone that is superior and inferior to the optic zone or by placing two raised areas with orientation cams at the 3 and 9 o'clock positions (Figure 7.4 (a) and (b)). No additional thickness is added to allow lens stabilization in the former design. The lids will squeeze against the thickness differential across the lens, maintaining its stability.

The advantage of this type of design is that the overall thickness profile can be kept to a minimum, optimizing physiological response

and patient comfort. A limitation of this design approach is that the resultant thickness differential is dependent on lens power. This results in a greater thickness differential for higher minus-powered lenses and therefore more effective stabilization.

In practical terms this may result in variable orientation between powers and emphasizes the need to trial lenses that closely match the patient's refractive error to allow accurate orientation assessment.

A recent refinement to this stabilization approach is a design that isolates the optical correction within an optic zone resulting in independent stabilization areas.[13] This allows orientation consistency across all powers and a thin overall thickness profile

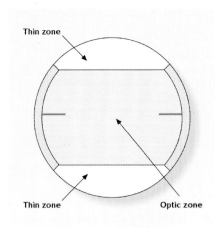

Figure 7.4(a)
An example of a dynamically stabilized lens from Grant.[9]

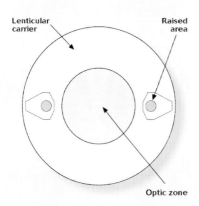

Figure 7.4(b)
An example of a dynamically stabilized lens, from Grant.[9]

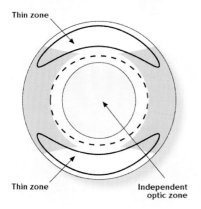

Figure 7.4(c)
Dynamic stabilization with independent optic zone to minimize stability inconsistency with different lens power, from Hickson–Curran et al.[13]

to improve oxygen transmissibility (Figure 7.4 (c)).

As no one soft toric design is suitable for all eyes, the practitioner should have a minimum of two designs available, to include both the prism-stabilized and dynamically stabilized design.

As well as having available soft toric lenses with different designs, the practitioner should also ensure the lenses being fitted are reproducible and, for non-disposable type lenses, that exchanges are available from the manufacturer, if required. Soft toric lens reproducibility, has improved over the years,[14] although lathe-cut lenses, in particular, might still show some variability.

All soft toric lenses require some form of marking on the lens by which the prac-

Cylinder power (D)	Percentage distribution of axis orientation in each cylinder power		
	With the rule	**Against the rule**	**Axis oblique**
0.50	36	34	30
1.00	34	34	32
1.50	35	31	34
2.00	38	24	38
2.50	50	18	32
3.00	54	17	29
3.50	49	17	34
4.00	50	15	35
Over 4.00	58	13	29

Table 7.2
Distribution of cylinder axis orientations, from Bennett.[1]

titioner can identify the position of the cylinder power axes. A variety of symbols are used by manufacturers to mark either the 6 o'clock or prism base of the lens or the 3 and 9 o'clock positions (Figures 7.5(a) and (b)).

Techniques

Initial fitting
The exact fitting procedures for soft toric lenses will vary from lens to lens. The basic principles, however, remain the same as long as a toric lens is used for on-eye assessment.

Some manufacturers advocate empirical fitting, i.e. ordering the final lens without first observing a lens on the eye and then making any adjustments that may be needed once the lens has been ordered. Disposable toric lens fitting allows an individual trial lens to be ordered empirically or the appropriate powered lens to be selected from an in-practice fitting bank.

Physical fit
The physical fit for a soft toric lens should be the same as for a spherical soft lens. The lens should cover the cornea in all the gaze positions, allow adequate tear flow to enable metabolic debris to be removed and remain in alignment to the cornea and conjunctiva.

If a lens fit is borderline between being adequate or having slight excessive movement, the more mobile fit would generally be chosen to allow lids to have the desired effect on the lens rotation.

Initial trial lens — choice and insertion
The choice of back optic zone radius (BOZR), total diameter (TD) and centre thickness (tc) for a soft toric lens should be made in the same way as one would select a spherical soft design. The power of the lens should be chosen with the spherical and, more importantly, the cylindrical power and axis as close as possible to the predicted final lens parameters. While earlier soft toric designs tended to predictably rotate nasally by 5–10 degrees, this is not usually the case with more modern designs and therefore no initial compensation of the cylindrical axis should be made when choosing the initial trial lens.

As both the cylinder power and axis is varied on a lens, there is a risk that different stability and degrees of rotations may result, especially with designs where the stabilizing thickness profile is dependent on lens power. Contrary to popular belief, axes of astigmatism are almost equally distributed around the clock face (Table 7.2). Oblique cylinders are generally accepted as being more difficult to achieve success with in terms of vision although more recent advanced designs attempt to minimize these rotational differences. The goal of the trial fitting is two-fold: to assess the physical fit and physiological response to the lens and to predict the lens rotation. Following insertion, the lens should be allowed to settle, as for a spherical soft lens, before the fit is assessed.

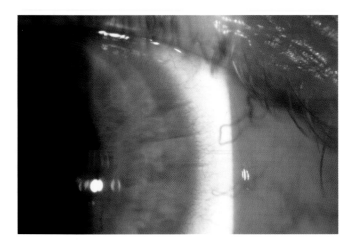

Figure 7.5(a)
Axis rotation marks on soft toric lenses.

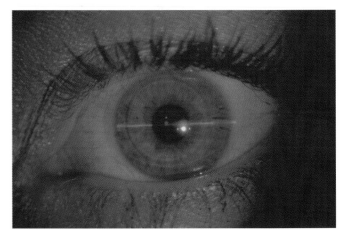

Figure 7.6
Slit-lamp rotation to measure lens position.

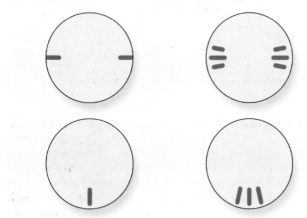

Figure 7.5(b)
Axis rotation marks on soft toric lenses.

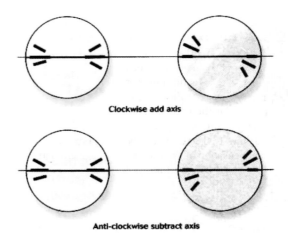

Figure 7.7
Examples showing alignment and misalignment of location marks.

Visual assessment

After this settling period, the patient should return to the practice and an over-refraction should be carried out. The purpose of the over-refraction is not to determine lens power or degree of rotation, but to see how stable the end-point result is and effectively assess lens stability. If the patient reports that the vision blurs with each blink, either the lens fit is unsuitable or the rotational stability of the lens is poor. In either case, another lens needs to be inserted, either a different parameter (in the case of a poor fit) or design (if the lens is rotationally unstable). Assuming that a clear end-point of refraction can be obtained, the practitioner should go on to assess the lens fit and rotational position.

Before the physical fit is determined, the practitioner should look first for the rotational stability of the lens. This is carried out by viewing the axis location marks on the lens. These should not show rotation with each blink and should be close to their intended position (vertically or horizontally). If the lens position is more than 30 degrees from the intended position it suggests that there is inadequate stabilization and an alternative lens design should be considered.

If the location marks are stable, the practitioner should note their position in relation to their intended position and the direction and degree of rotation seen (if any). This can either be measured using a graticule, the slit-beam rotation on the slit-lamp (Figure 7.6) or estimated using the axis marks as a guide (Figure 7.7).

The axis rotation gives the practitioner the information needed to order the next lens. The rotation of the lens shows how far the axis of the cylinder will be mislocated when the final lens is placed on the eye. This mislocation can be compensated for by ordering a lens with the axis at a different position.

If, for example, an ocular refraction is $-3.00/-1.75 \times 180$ and a trial lens rotates clockwise by 10 degrees when placed on the eye, the correction will be $-3.00/-1.75 \times 170$ degrees and the vision will be blurred. To compensate for this, if the lenses are ordered as $-3.00/-1.75 \times 10$, the 10 degree clockwise rotation will bring the axis round to 180 degrees, the required axis, and vision will be clear. Note that the location marks should still be observed at 10 degrees clockwise.

The basic rule is that if the lens rotates clockwise the degree of rotation should be added to the axis, but if it rotates anticlockwise the rotation should be subtracted from the axis (CAAS). Alternatively, if the lens rotates to the left the rotation should be added and if it is to the right it should be subtracted (LARS).

Over-refraction

If the trial lens scribe marks lie within 10 degrees of the intended position, vision can be assessed and a spherical over-refraction carried out to determine whether an alternate spherical power should be ordered. Lenses that position off-axis will produce a residual refractive error which is a function of the cylinder power and degree of mis-orientation. For example, a toric soft lens of power $-3.00/-1.75 \times 180$ that matches the patient's ocular prescription but orientates 20 degrees off-axis will result in an over-refraction of $+0.60/-1.20 \times 55$. The stability of the end-point gives a good indication that lens fit is adequate, however it is difficult to determine whether the spherical component of the final prescription to be ordered requires adjustment. Consequently, a new trial lens should be inserted after compensation of the cylinder axis for lens rotation to allow a meaningful spherical over-refraction.

The final order for the lens should include BOZR, TD, tc (if variable) and the power in terms of the sphere, cylinder and desired axis.

Troubleshooting: poor vision

The most common problem encountered with soft toric lens fitting is unacceptable visual acuity. The most common reason for this is mis-location of the axis. The visual acuity might be found to be reduced, either at the time of dispensing, with the final lens or at a subsequent aftercare examination.

If poor vision is found at dispensing, the practitioner should first review the patient's record to see what the power of the trial lens was. If the power of the trial lens (spherical and axis) was similar to that of the prescription lens, one or other of the lenses might differ from the marked parameters. In some cases, the reason for the poor vision is axis rotation caused by the different effects of the eyelid on the final prescription lens and on the trial lens. This in turn can be brought on by the different thickness profiles, and therefore stabilization effectiveness, of some lens designs. This problem can be avoided by using trial lenses

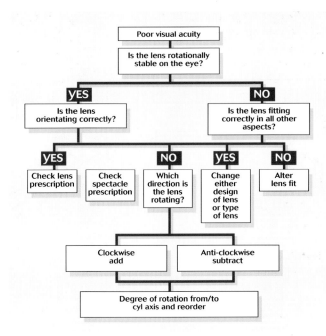

Figure 7.8
Flowchart procedure to approach the problem of poor visual acuity

that closely match the patient's ocular prescription or using lens designs that offer independent optical and stabilization areas.

Figure 7.8 suggests a flowchart procedure to tackle poor visual acuity.[15] This approach is based on assessing the rotational stability of the lens in the eye. If the lens is rotationally stable but the axis is mis-located, the practitioner compensates for axis rotation and reorders the lens. If the lens is rotationally unstable, either a different fit or design of the soft toric lens is required.

An alternative procedure is to record the over-refraction and then calculate the power of the new lens using the formula for crossed cylinders. The problems with this are two fold: in many cases, the prescribing practitioner merely supplies the values to the manufacturer and awaits a new lens. When this happens, the practitioner is effectively losing control of the procedure. The second problem is that the calculation for the new lens might result in a larger cylinder power than the original prescription. As cylinder power is one of the determinants of lens rotation with some designs, the lens might become even more rotationally unstable. It is preferable to address the initial cause of the problem by compensating directly for axis rotation.

However, a sphere/cyl over-refraction can be useful in determining whether poor visual acuity is due to lens mis-location alone or resulting from differences between labelled and actual specification. If the residual refractive error shows a result where the cylinder power is numerically twice the sphere power, it is a good indication that the lens is simply sitting off-axis.[16]

A survey by Remba[17] showed that an average of 1.8 lenses per eye was required to achieve a successful result when fitting toric lenses. Other studies have shown findings of 1.5 lenses per eye to achieve a successful fit.

Troubleshooting: poor comfort

Lens comfort has been shown to be related to overall lens volume. If a patient is complaining of comfort problems with soft toric lenses, the practitioner should consider changing the design of the lens to one that has a thinner profile. This can be achieved, for example, by moving to a thinner prism stabilized design or from a prism stabilized design to a dynamically stabilized lens.

Troubleshooting: oedema

The increased thickness of soft toric lenses over spherical soft lenses means there is less oxygen transmission to the eye, which in turn can result in localized oedema.

Early toric lens designs with low water content and increased thickness profiles did produce significant corneal oedema.

To increase oxygen flow, the practitioner should either use a design with a thinner profile or higher water content or ideally a combination of both. More modern designs address this issue by using the minimum bulk to achieve stability. Thin, mid-water content dynamic stabilization designs have been shown to offer the highest overall transmissibility.[13]

Troubleshooting: staining

As soft torics are specifically designed to prevent rotation to achieve the desired optical effect, this might result in reduced tear exchange and entrapment of debris. In turn, this can result in corneal staining. If corneal staining occurs, the same principles for its management apply for soft toric lenses as for soft spherical lenses.

Key points

- Improvements in toric lens stability, oxygen transmissibility and reproducibility mean that practitioners should be confident in fitting soft toric lenses when poor vision is due to astigmatism.
- Assessing rotational stability is the key to success.
- Practitioners should have a variety of lens designs to choose from which include prism and dynamic stabilization designs.
- Practitioners should allow for more than one lens per eye, both in terms of time and financial consideration, but only attempt a maximum of three lenses per eye.

Summary

Over thirty per cent of prescriptions have 0.75D or greater of refractive astigmatism, although only approximately 16 per cent of all soft lenses fitted are torics. Of the strategies to correct astigmatism with soft contact lenses, the use of the soft toric lens provides the least compromised means. Soft toric fitting has become simpler in recent years and manufacturing technology has improved so that soft torics

should become an integral part of contact lens practice.

Question 7.1
Approximately what percentage of prescriptions have 0.75DC or more of ocular astigmatism?
  A 20 per cent
  B 10 per cent
  C 16 per cent
  D 33 per cent
  E 5 per cent

Question 7.2
Which of the following cannot be used to correct an astigmatic refractive error in the majority of cases?
  A Aspheric RGP
  B Toric periphery
  C Spherical RGP
  D Bi-toric RGP
  E Spherical soft

Question 7.3
What area of a prism-stabilized soft toric lens is the thinnest?
  A Centre
  B Superior
  C Inferior
  D Nasal
  E Temporal

Question 7.4
Which area of a dynamic stabilized soft toric lens is the thinnest?
  A Centre
  B Superior and inferior
  C Inferior
  D Superior
  E Temporal and nasal

Question 7.5
Successful toric soft lens fitting requires:
  A No lens movement
  B Rotational stability
  C Thinner lens design
  D Smaller TD
  E Excessive lens movement

Question 7.6
Orientation of a soft toric contact lens does not rely on:
  A Lid/lens interaction
  B Lens power
  C Lens thickness profile
  D Gravity
  E Overall fit

Question 7.7
Axes of astigmatism less than 2.00DC are distributed:
  A Almost equally around the clock face
  B More commonly 'with the rule'
  C More commonly 'against the rule'
  D More commonly with oblique axes
  E Predominantly associated 'with and against' the rule

Question 7.8
Axes of astigmatism greater than 2.50DC are distributed:
  A Almost equally around the clock face
  B More commonly 'with the rule'
  C More commonly 'against the rule'
  D More commonly with oblique axes
  E Predominantly associated 'with and against' the rule

Question 7.9
A spectacle refraction is found to be, $-6.00/-2.25 \times 10$ at vertex distance 10 mm. What lens power would you initially trial?
  A $-6.00/-2.25 \times 10$
  B $-5.75/-2.00 \times 10$
  C $-5.50/-2.25 \times 10$
  D $-5.75/-1.75 \times 10$
  E $-5.50/-1.75 \times 10$

Question 7.10
An ocular refraction is found to be $-2.00/-1.75 \times 180°$. A trial lens placed on the eye rotates anticlockwise by $10°$. What lens prescription would you order to compensate for this?
  A $-2.00/-1.75 \times 180°$
  B $-2.00/-1.75 \times 10°$
  C $-2.00/-1.75 \times 170°$
  D $-2.00/-1.75 \times 90°$
  E $-2.00/-1.75 \times 80°$

References

1 Bennett, A.G. and Rabbetts, R.B. (1984) Distribution and ocular dioptrics of ametropia. In: *Clinical Visual Optics* Butterworth-Heinemann, 433–434.

2 Edwards, K. and Hough, T. (1994) Toric periphery rigid lenses. *JBCLA* **17:4** 107–114.

3 Meyler, J. and Ruston, D. (1995) Toric RGP contact lenses made easy. *Optician* **209:5504** 30–35.

4 Meyler, J. and Morgan, P. (1997) Advanced contact lens fitting. Part 2. Toric rigid lens fitting. *Optician* **5604:213** 18–23.

5 Grant, R. (1986) The elliptical fitting philosophy: hard gas-permeable lenses. *Optician* **191:5032** 24–31.

6 Harris, M.G. *et al.* (1995) Do disposable contact lenses mask astigmatism? *CL Spectrum* **10:6** 21–28.

7 Lydon, D. (1990) Improved optics and control of astigmatism without cylinders. *BCLA Trans* 41–43.

8 Killpartrick, M. (1983) Apples, space-time and the watermelon seed. *Optician* **186:4823** 801–802.

9 Grant, R. (1995) Toric soft contact lenses: a review. *Optician* **209:5483** 16–24.

10 Tanner, J. (1996) A new high water content soft toric lens. *Optician* **211:5549** 20–21.

11 Ruston, D. (1999) Success with soft torics and high astigmats: the Hydrasoft Toric. *Optician* **217:5704** 34–38.

12 Cox, I., Comstock, T. and Reindel, W. (1999) A clinical comparison of two soft toric contact lenses. *Optician* **218:5730** 32–36.

13 Hickson-Curran, S., Veys, J. and Dalton, L. (2000) A new dual-thin zone disposable toric lens. *Optician* **219:5736** 18–26.

14 Davies, I.P (1990) A comparison of the reproducibility of soft toric contact lenses. *CL Spectrum* **5:10** 79–82.

15 Davies, I.P. (1989) Soft toric contact lenses: systematic approach to problem-solving *Optician* **198:5211** 16–18.

16 Edwards, K. (1999) Problem solving with toric soft contact lenses. *Optician* **217:5695** 18–27.

17 Remba, M. (1986) Clinical evaluation of soft toric contact lenses. *Optician* **192:5066** 17–24.

8
Managing the presbyope

Introduction

As the number of patients wearing contact lenses around the world grows, so does the number requiring presbyopic correction. Patients fitted with lenses in the 1970s are now beginning to experience presbyopia and demand satisfactory correction without recourse to spectacles.

There is also the demand from presbyopic hyperopes who, on reaching presbyopia, now need full-time correction for distance and near and, with more active lifestyles and increased awareness of contact lenses, are asking for contact lens correction. The number of presbyopic patients in Europe is on a steady incline and is forecast to grow further over the next five years (Figure 8.1). Practitioners can therefore expect to see an increase in the number of presbyopes attending for contact lens fittings over the next few years.

As the size of the presbyopic market increases, so too does the number of options for correcting presbyopia with contact lenses. The history of contact lens correction of presbyopia has been one of products being launched onto the market with claims that have never been realized in practice. This has lead to scepticism by practitioners about claims made by the industry and a reluctance to fully embrace some of the products launched. Before looking at the techniques required to correct presbyopia with contact lenses, we should first review some of the options as shown in Figure 8.2.

Spectacles

Probably the most common method of correcting the contact lens-wearing presbyope is with a pair of reading spectacles worn over the distance contact lens correction. These may either be full-frame single vision, multifocal or a half-eye depending on the needs of the individual. Such correction puts the presbyopic contact lens wearer in the same category as the presbyopic emmetrope. The advantage of this technique is that the contact lens correction requires no modifications which, assuming that it is optimum at the time of fitting, remains the case

The obvious disadvantage is, of course, that the principal reason for contact lens wear is being ignored. Contact lens patients do not want to wear spectacles, because, if they did, they would be doing so already. Consequently, pure contact lens options should be explained first to the presbyopic contact lens wearers, followed by the spectacle correction option if appropriate.

Monovision

Monovision is the correction of one eye with the distance prescription and the contra-lateral eye with the near prescription. It works on the principle that the visual system can suppress the central focus image and thus enable the object of interest to be seen clearly. Monovision remains an effective means of correcting presbyopia with contact lenses, and, as such, an understanding of its indications and contraindications is essential to the practitioner dealing with presbyopic patients.

Monovision clearly disrupts a patient's stereopsis and, for some patients who have either little tolerance for visual disruption or who are engaged in detailed visual tasks, this disruption might prove too great. While some investigators have tried to develop predictive tests to assess which patients might prove suitable for monovision, these have not proved to be as valuable as simply allowing the patient to try the lenses. An advantage of monovision is that it allows the practitioner to choose the most suitable lens for the patient (such as the material type and design) without having to add the compromise that might exist with a particular bifocal design (for example, limited oxygen transmissibility).

Whenever monovision has been compared directly with bifocal or multifocal contact lenses in controlled clinical trials, monovision has had a success rate equal to, or above that, of the bifocal in question (Figure 8.3). In addition, the less compromised near visual acuity performance in all illuminations provided by monovision is an indication for consideration of this type of fitting option for presbyopes with strong near vision demands. However, when critical or sustained tasks requiring good distance binocularity predominate, it is advisable to avoid monovision or to consider supplementary correction. A more recent study by Dutoit et al[7] has shown that adapted monovision wearers rated many aspects of subjective vision performance higher with simultaneous vision bifocal

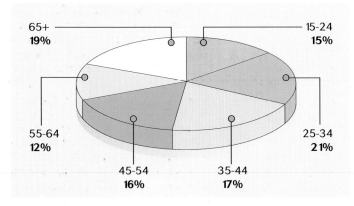

Figure 8.1
UK demographics, 1997, showing 47 per cent of the population over the age of 45.

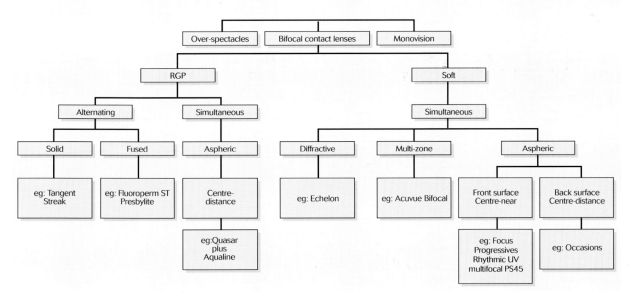

Figure 8.2 *Contact lens options for presbyopes*

contact lenses. These included distance vision in good and poor lighting, driving at night and depth perception. Near vision in poor lighting was rated higher during monovision wear.

Alternating bifocals

The alternating, or translating bifocal, was one of the first types of bifocal contact lenses to be produced. The patient looks through the distance portion of the optic zone in primary gaze (Figure 8.4). On down gaze, the lens is held up against the lower eyelid, so the visual axis looks through the near portion. The advantage is that visual quality will remain high as long as the visual axis is directed through the appropriate part of the lens. The disadvantage is that, for this to occur, significant eyelid/lens interaction needs to occur, which can lead to decreased patient comfort through increased lens bulk and mobility.

Attempts to produce translating bifocals in soft designs have generally proved unsuccessful. In rigid lens materials, the challenge is to produce a lens with a different-powered near portion while maintaining a smooth passage of the upper eyelid over the anterior surface. The two distinct portions that make up an alternating lens may be either fused or solid portions with a range of alternative segment shapes (Figure 8.5). Prism, truncation or both control lens stability, position and translation.

Simultaneous vision designs

Simultaneous vision bifocals rely on an optical system that places two images on the retina simultaneously and then relies on the visual system to 'select' the clearer picture (versus monovision in which a clear image is placed on each retina, the confusion occurring at a higher part of the visual pathway). Early simultaneous vision bifocals had discrete zones of distance and near vision (Figures 8.6(a) and (b)). In more recent designs, the power distribution across the lens surface has been variable and lenses have been described as multifocal, aspheric or progressive (Figures 8.7(a) and (b)) and are available in both soft and rigid materials. Alternatively, lens designs can consist of a number of concentric zones to control visual performance in varying illumination levels (Figure 8.8) or involve a combination of diffractive and refractive optics to achieve bifocal correction (Figure 8.9).

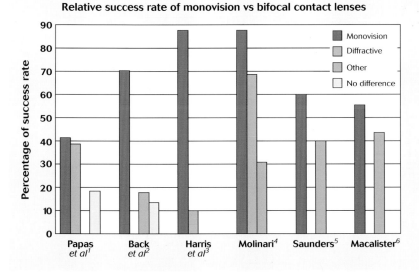

Figure 8.3
Comparison of success rates of monovision with a variety of different bifocal contact lenses.

Aspheric centre-distance

A centre-distance lens usually has a back-

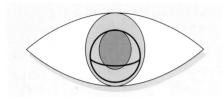
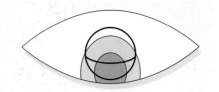

Figure 8.4
The principle of the translating bifocal contact.

surface aspheric curve resulting in the central portion of its optical zone for distance vision, which is surrounded by an area containing the power of lens required for near work. This is achieved by the aspheric curve inducing positive spherical aberration. Rays of light from a distant object are focused by the central zone on the retina and compete with the out-of-focus rays being formed by the surround (Figure 8.10). When regarding a near object, the reverse occurs, and this time it is the light rays from the peripheral zone that come into focus. The visual system then picks out the clearer of the two images.

The greater the eccentricity (or rate of flattening) of the back surface aspheric curve the higher the reading power in relation to distance power. However, the higher the reading addition, the more likely that distance vision will be affected adversely, especially in low contrast and/or low light conditions. Current back surface aspheric soft lenses are therefore recommended for early presbyopia only (up to +1.25D). In soft lenses, the aspheric back surface will not normally have any significant impact on fit, but in rigid gas-permeable lenses the back surface geometry may depart significantly from corneal

topography. This is due to rapidly flattening back surface aspheric geometry and will be fitted significantly steeper to allow appropriate lens centration.[9] Back surface aspheric RGP lens designs can now be based on corneal topography and ocular prescription to create an individual lens design for correcting presbyopia.[10] The aim is to modify the combined optical system of the lens, tears and cornea to provide a predictable multifocal effect.

Probably the most fundamental concern with such a system is in its dependency on the pupil size. The near pupil reactions mean that, as a near object is brought into view proportionally, less of the pupil allows light in from the near zone of the lens.

Aspheric centre-near
Centre-near bifocal and aspheric designs were introduced to address the problem of pupil constriction for close work. The optical principle is the same as for the centre-distance lens, although reversed, so this time it is the central portion of the lens that forms the light from close objects and is surrounded by the required distance power (Figure 8.11). Front surface soft aspheric designs promote negative spherical aber-

ration and the aspheric curve can be calculated to limit the spherical aberrations of the eye and, if necessary, of the lens itself. The improvement of retinal image quality and increase in depth of focus can be effective at correcting the early presbyope (up to +1.50D). Apart from the visual demands of the presbyope, it would also be expected that visual performance would depend upon the interaction of the optical characteristics of the particular lens design with the aberrations of the eyes of the wearer. Consequently, variations in ocular aberration between individuals may explain in part why lenses of this type meet the needs of some wearers but not others.[11] As presbyopia increases, correcting the wearers' spherical aberration alone will not be sufficient and the front surface curve must have a greater degree of asphericity to allow more plus refractive power within the optical system. This often involves more complex surface geometry of varying eccentricity to allow stabilized distance and near power zones within a specified area which is design dependent.

Multi-zone concentric centre-distance
It became clear that with future designs, greater attention should be paid to minimizing the dependency of lens function on pupil size, especially in relation to different lighting conditions. One approach is to increase the number of concentric zones alternatively powered for distance and near vision. This concept resulted in a centre-distance multi-zone design consisting of five alternating distance and near powered zones (see Figure 8.8). The width and

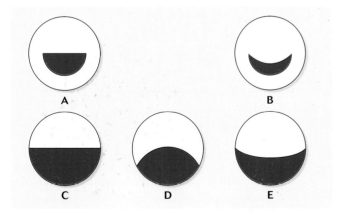
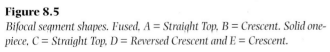

Figure 8.5
Bifocal segment shapes. Fused, A = Straight Top, B = Crescent. Solid one-piece, C = Straight Top, D = Reversed Crescent and E = Crescent.

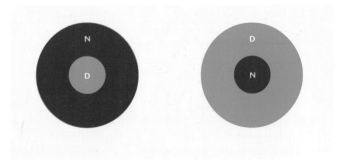

Figure 8.6
Bi-concentric centre-distance design (left). Bi-concentric centre near-design (right).

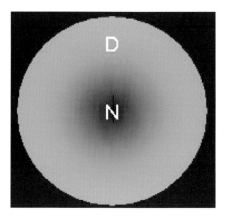

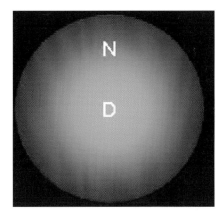

Figure 8.7
Front surface centre-near design (left). Back surface centre-distance design (right).

spacing of the zones is based on the variation of pupil size in different illuminations within the presbyopic population. Theoretically, the lens design favours distance vision in extreme high and low lighting conditions and provides a more equal ratio of light division in ambient illumination conditions.[12] The multiple ring configuration is designed to provide vision which is more specific to the available lighting conditions. Transition curves between the concentric zones are such that the zones are not readily visible on the slit-lamp biomicroscope.

Diffractive bifocals

Diffractive lenses work on the principle of placing a phase plate on the rear surface of the lens, which is able to split the light passing through into two discrete focal points, one for distance and the other for near vision (see Figure 8.9). The performance of the lenses, therefore, becomes independent of pupil size as long as the pupil diameter remains smaller than the diffractive zone in the lens. The disadvantages of diffractive lenses are two-fold. While not pupil size dependent, they are centration dependent and their performance decreases as the lens decentres. They also significantly reduce the contrast of an object, which is a factor of diffractive optics. This makes this type of lens less suitable for detailed visual tasks in low illumination environments.

Instrumentation

The basic instrumentation required for presbyopic contact lens fitting is the same as that needed to fit regular rigid gaspermeable or soft contact lenses.

Lens trial

It is essential to be able to trial a lens, regardless of the design, which is as close as possible to the patient's refractive needs. This can be ordered empirically or, ideally, be made available from in-practice single-use fitting banks. This allows a more realistic assessment by the patient and practitioner as well as allowing vision assessment in the work and home environment. To assess the outcome of a fit, the patient has to experience vision as it will be in the final lens. Judging success simply by measuring acuity alone will not provide an effective predictor of outcome.

Visual assessment

As indicated above, the assessment of visual acuity alone is a poor indicator of success with presbyopic (and indeed much non-presbyopic) contact lens practice. Practitioners must have tools available to help both themselves and patients judge the visual performance. High and low contrast visual acuity charts (Figure 8.12) give more information about acuity and, in particular, the difference in low-contrast acuity between spectacles and contact lenses gives some indication of possible success.

As well as the visual acuity charts, the practitioner should have access to other near tasks, such as the opportunity to sit patients at an office desk viewing a VDU screen (possibly in the reception area) and a wide variety of different coloured paper and contrasts of type. Needles, threads, screws, nuts and bolts can also provide useful visual props in helping to assess visual performance.

Lighting

Lighting plays an important part in seeing, particularly in assessing vision for the presbyope. Ideally, the consulting room should have a wide range of lighting possibilities. These should range from bright, direct illumination on targets to maximize the chances of a patient first seeing the in-focus image, through to the ability to decrease the level of illumination so visual performance at, or near, darkness can be assessed. It might also be valuable to have a glare source on, or near, visual tasks to help in assessing the effect of glare on vision.

Techniques

The techniques for correcting presbyopia with contact lenses will vary from lens type to lens type. There are, however, certain fundamental principles in presbyopic correction that will be discussed in detail in this

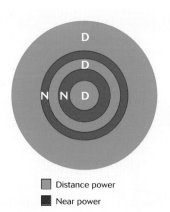

Distance power
Near power

Figure 8.8
Multi-zone concentric centre-distance design.

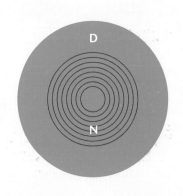

Figure 8.9
Diffractive design.

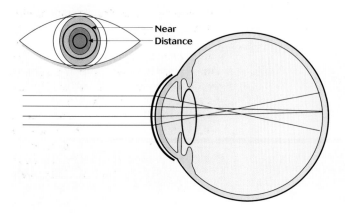

Figure 8.10
Principle of simultaneous vision centre-distance design.

chapter, with reference to the type of correction being made. The reader is referred to individual manufacturers' fitting guides for more details. As with all contact lens fitting, the practitioner must ensure the patient is suitable to wear lenses. As the eye ages, a number of conditions might affect this suitability that have to be taken into account. It is also important that the patient is given realistic expectations about the likely level of vision and the compromises that are inherent in this type of contact lens correction. This involves discussing the benefits of combined distance/near correction without the need for spectacles as well as likely differences between the visual performance of monovision, simultaneous or alternating vision lenses. When compared to spectacles or single-vision contact lenses, this may take the form of reductions in visual acuity, especially in low luminance, stereopsis and reduced intermediate vision depending on the type of lens fitted. It is also an opportunity to explain to the patient that it is quite normal that fitting requires more than one appointment to trial alternative lens powers and fitting approaches.

Monovision

Physical fit
The physical and physiological fit of a contact lens required to correct presbyopes by the monovision technique will be the same as the fit required by one used without modification.

Ocular dominance
Monovision works because the visual system is able to suppress the blurred foveal image in an eye. In general, the visual system is better able to suppress an image in the non-dominant rather than the dominant eye, and it is for this reason that ocular dominance should be assessed. An empirical means of assessing ocular dominance is to ask patients if they are right or left handed and assume that ocular follows motor dominance. While this is true in many cases, there are some in which the reverse is true and others for which there is no strong dominance, a valuable finding in itself.

Alternative and preferred means of assessing ocular dominance include 'pointing' and 'sighting'. In the former, patients are asked to clasp their hands together with forefingers pointing out like a child pretending to fire a gun. They are then asked to keep their eyes open and to point the fingers at one of the practitioner's eyes, with the practitioner sitting at the opposite end of the room. The practitioner then looks to see which of the patient's eyes the fingers are lined up with – this is the dominant eye.

In sighting, the patient holds a card with a hole at arm's length, with the practitioner asking him or her to view a distant object. Once the object is sighted, the practitioner again looks to see which of the patient's eyes is lined up with the object. This is the dominant eye.

An alternative approach to preferential looking is termed the +2.00D blur test. This involves placing the best binocular distance refraction in the trial frame and, while the patient looks at the lowest line they can read, a +2.00D is placed alternatively in front of each eye. The patient indicates when the vision is clearest. If the +2.00D lens is in front of the left eye when the image is reported as clearest then the right eye is considered as distance dominant and vice versa. It has been found that unsuccessful wearers became successful after switching near and distance corrections contrary to the dominance as measured by traditional methods but rarely contrary to the +2.00D test.[13]

Trial lens power selection
For the majority of patients, a good starting point in selecting appropriate lens power is to fit the dominant eye with the distance correction and then the non-dominant eye with the full-near correction. It is also recommended that the practitioner should, at this stage, avoid going into the detailed mechanics of how the vision is being corrected. It is important to correct any astigmatism equal to or greater than 0.75D in either or both eyes which, if left uncorrected, can result in reduced visual

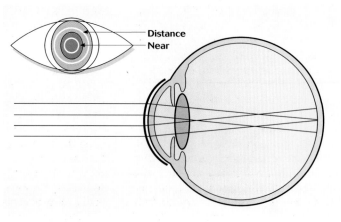

Figure 8.11
Principle of simultaneous vision centre-near design.

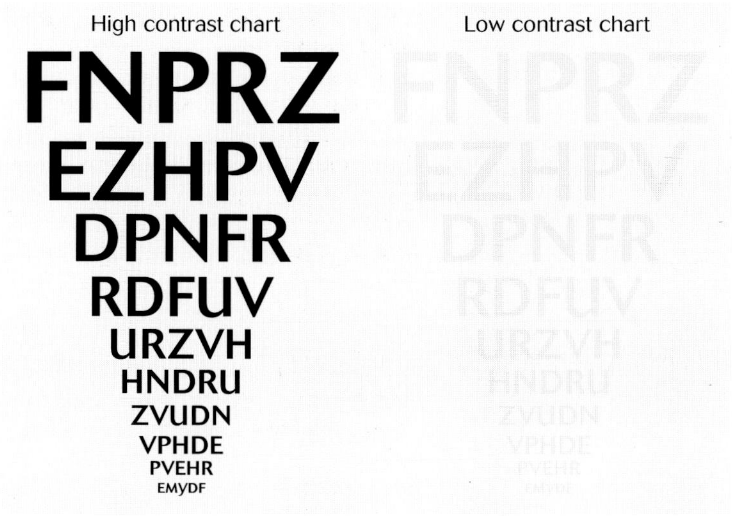

High contrast chart

Low contrast chart

FNPRZ
EZHPV
DPNFR
RDFUV
URZVH
HNDRU
ZVUDN
VPHDE
PVEHR
EMYDF

Figure 8.12
High and low contrast visual acuity chart.

performance acuity, asthenopic symptoms and poor tolerance.

Visual assessment
The first task for the practitioner is to encourage the patient to suppress each eye to see clearly. The ability to do this occurs at a subconscious level, so the practitioner should not immediately explain how the vision has been corrected. Under binocular viewing, looking at a high-contrast, well-illuminated distance chart, the patient should be asked to read as far down the chart as possible without comment on visual quality. The patient should then be directed towards a high-contrast near type, with illumination again being high to maximize the chances of seeing the image. Once again, the patient should be asked to read as far as possible. If they are unable to read with the distance or the near type, the practitioner should not, at this stage, occlude either eye. Instead, the 'non- viewing eye' in the situation that has the out-of-focus image should be progressively blurred with spherical lenses until the image comes into view.

When the distance or near type is seen clearly, the amount of blur should be progressively reduced while asking the patient to continue to read. Once the full extent of the blur has been removed, the patient should be asked to view a distant object (if it was the near test that was causing problems before) and then return to reading. This technique will demonstrate the ability of the patient to suppress the 'non-viewing' eye.

Once the ability to suppress has been demonstrated, the practitioner should optimize the refraction, again binocularly to check that the optimum correction for distance and near has been achieved. It is only then that the practitioner should explain to the patient how the vision has been corrected. The maxim 'show then tell' is probably one of the key factors behind success in monovision fitting.

After static visual acuity has been assessed, the patient should be encouraged to walk around the practice wearing the full monovision correction. It is here that the use of free trial disposable or frequent replacement lenses is of value in allowing the exact prescription to be fitted and trialled. The dynamic visual assessment should start with an appreciation of the effect of suppression on peripheral acuity before allowing the patient to carry out other tasks, such as judging distance. These assessments are important, both clinically and ethically, in showing the patient the advantages and limitations of the correction.

Ideally, an extended trial period is preferred in monovision correction so that the patient can fully assess the benefits of the correction. Before this occurs, the onus is on the practitioner to explain fully the type of correction fitted and to make sure the patient understands that the adaptation period may involve problems in close work and a 'learning curve' in driving, especially at night. For most road users, monovision still provides adequate visual performance to meet regulatory standards, although the EU directive on driving licences requires that a driver of a Grade 2 vehicle (greater than 750 kilograms) must have a minimum of 6/12 vision in the worst eye. When fitting monovision, and indeed all presbyopic contact lens corrections, the practitioner has an obligation to inform patients of the adaptation that may be required. If a patient is unable to adapt to any visual disturbance caused by monovision in specific situations, a practitioner may consider prescribing a spectacle over-refraction.

Partial monovision
Generally the acceptance, and therefore the success of monovision, falls as the reading add increases.[14,15] As the indicated add exceeds +2.00D, tolerance can often be improved if a reduced reading addition is given. The patient may need 'top up' glasses for small print and possibly additional glasses for driving, or a secondary distance-correcting contact lens. This form of monovision is ideal for social users whose near vision demands will be lower than full-time wearers. It is also useful for patients who have greater intermediate vision needs.

Enhanced monovision fitting
Enhanced monovision involves fitting one eye with a bifocal lens and the other with a single vision lens. A variety of options exist. The more frequent approach involves fitting the dominant eye with a single-vision distance lens (spherical or toric) and the non-dominant eye with a bifocal lens. This improves binocular summation and offers some level of stereo-acuity to the monovision wearer that is experiencing increasing blur with a higher reading add. Alternatively the same approach can be used when fitting patients that require sharper distance vision than bilateral simultaneous vision can offer. The bifocal lens in the non-dominant eye usually needs more bias for near. This modification can be achieved effectively by increasing the distance power of the bifocal lens by +0.50D to +0.75D while reducing the add power accordingly.

Alternating vision bifocals
Physical fit
An alternating vision rigid bifocal must be fitted to allow translation between the distance and near zone to occur. The lens should, therefore, be mobile and supported by the lower eye-lid. In primary gaze, the

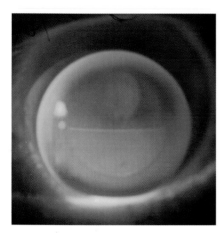

Figure 8.13(a)
Segment position in primary position of gaze (courtesy of David Ruston).

lower pupil margin should be in line with the top of the near segment (Figure 8.13(a)). On near vision, the pupil should look through the near segment (Figure 8.13(b)). The fit is most effectively assessed by using a hand-held Burton lamp and fluorescein. The hand-held Burton lamp is preferable to the slit-lamp as it encourages a more natural head posture. If the lens does not centre adequately, the fit should be modified.

Trial lens power selection
Once the lens fit has been optimized, a normal binocular over-refraction should be carried out at both distance and near. The use of a trial frame and lenses is preferred to the refractor head as it allows a more natural head posture, which is critical in fitting this type of lens. The practitioner should avoid any consideration of over-plussing the prescription during the refraction. Alternating bifocals are designed to function by having two discrete focal lengths for distance and near. If the only way of achieving a satisfactory result is to dramatically alter the binocular refractive state, the lenses are not being allowed to work in this way and lens translation should be improved or the practitioner should try a straight monovision correction.

Visual assessment
The static visual assessment is carried out in a similar way to monovision. It is, however, probable that a trial frame will have to be worn to provide the correct near refraction. Once again, visual contrast and illumination should remain high to assist the patient in visualizing the two images.

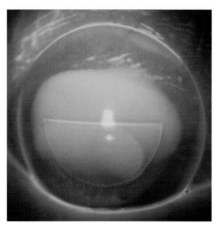

Figure 8.13(b)
Segment position positioned over pupil in down gaze due to successful lens translation (courtesy of David Ruston).

When assessing dynamic visual performance, the practitioner should demonstrate to the patient the effect of the near addition leading to an area of blur inferiority. As a patient new to bifocal or varifocal spectacles would be instructed, so the alternating vision bifocal contact lens wearer should be aware of this, although this effect will be less than with a spectacle lens due to the reduced vertex distance.

Simultaneous vision bifocals
Physical fit
In contrast to the alternating vision lens, the refractive optic simultaneous vision bifocal should be fitted with minimum, rather than maximum, movement. It is critical that the lens is well centred over the visual axis to enable the correct portion of light to pass through each part of the lens. As the lens decentres, the aberrations increase, to the detriment of vision. The optimum centration should not be achieved to the detriment of the physiological fit of the lens, and the squeeze pressure under the lens should be sufficient to allow tear exchange to occur.

Trial lens power selection
It is in power selection that simultaneous vision bifocals differ to the greatest extent, with different manufacturers recommending different strategies for varying designs. The basic principle in achieving correction is to provide a full binocular correction at distance and near. If the lens is working as a true bifocal, the distance correction should be determined first and the different near additions tested in turn. When assessing

distance correction, care should be taken to maximize the plus power of the lens to fully relax binocular accommodation. Although the most effective adjustment options may vary with the lens design being used, most designs are sensitive to 0.25 dioptre adjustments to the distance lens power which can have a profound effect on distance or near visual performance. Lens power adjustments are best investigated by using +/−0.25D twirls/flippers or trial lenses during binocular vision in ambient illumination, or the illumination where problems are being experienced by the wearer. The use of phoropters should be avoided during over-refraction as the resulting light reduction will increase pupil size and alter optical performance. Any distance minus power adjustment should only be made if it has been demonstrated to make a significant impact on distance visual acuity (i.e. half to one line of Snellen visual acuity) combined with a subjective improvement.

If a satisfactory distance and near correction cannot be achieved, many manufacturers recommend moving towards a 'modified monovision' technique by over-correcting one eye and under-correcting the other. This requires the assessment of ocular dominance and binocular variation to the prescription, as in monovision. The modified approach can be achieved by adjusting the refractive power of the lens or selecting alternative lens designs for each eye to deliberately improve distance vision in one eye, at the expense of near performance, while improving near in the other. This can be achieved by increasing the minus/decreasing the plus on the dominant eye to enhance distance vision, while decreasing the minus/increasing the plus in the non-dominant eye.

A similar bias can be obtained by using different add powers in each, the lower add power being fitted to the dominant eye to improve distance vision. Similarly, one eye may be fitted with a centre-distance simultaneous design and the other with a centre-near design, although with aspheric centre-near designs it is not always true that near performance is better than distance.

Visual assessment
Visual assessment, both static and dynamic, should be carried out as previously described. Particular note should be made of the effect of pupil size on visual

Grade	Descriptor	Description
5	Excellent	Sharp and clear at all times
4	Good	Occasional periods of blur
3	Satisfactory	Acceptable but slight blur/haze
2	Fair	Blur/haze noticeable at all times
1	Poor	Significant blur, unacceptable

Table 8.1
Visual quality assessment scale.

performance, which should be adequately explained to the patient.

Diffractive bifocals
Physical fit
A diffractive bifocal should show the same fitting characteristics as other simultaneous vision designs in that the phase plate must be centred over the visual axis in all positions of gaze.

Trial lens power selection
As with a simultaneous vision lens, the trial lens should be chosen as near as possible to the distance prescription, choosing the median near addition. Once again, a full binocular distance refraction should be carried out without regard to eye dominance. When the distance correction has been optimized, the patient should be asked to read some near print. It is important that the near print has a high contrast and is illuminated. If the print is not seen at first, the practitioner should avoid the temptation to increase the plus power.

Diffractive bifocals have two discrete foci, one for distance and the other for near. The page of near type should first be moved away and then towards the patient to see if it comes into clear vision. Once a clear point is found, the practitioner can try to use different over-corrections, which will probably necessitate changing the reading distance. The over-refraction required to see clearly for near type should neither exceed the near addition, nor blur the distance acuity. If it does, the distance portion of the lens is being used, not the near portion. In some cases, the patient may comment that the near print appears to 'jump out from the page'. This is a function of the clear image overlying the blurred distance image on the retina.

Visual assessment
This is carried out in the same way as for a simultaneous vision lens. The reduction in image contrast created by the diffractive lens should be demonstrated to the patient by decreasing the illumination of the near type. Patients should also be cautioned about the glare and flare they will experience when driving at night with a diffractive lens.

Troubleshooting: poor vision
The most common problem in presbyopic lens correction is inadequate vision. Although the visual acuity might be excellent, the patient could still complain of unacceptable vision because visual quality is not the same as visual acuity and with many correction options it is unlikely that objective and subjective visual performance will be the same as that experienced through a spectacle correction. Subjective assessment of visual quality, such as a 0–5 scale (Table 8.1) might help in recording this. If the visual quality is unacceptable, the first step should be to modify the refraction, which is most effectively achieved by placing trial lenses over the patient's eyes and ensuring that whatever improvement is made at one distance is not offset by significant degradation at another. If a lens type is to be changed, the practitioner should only consider switching from one basic principle to another and avoid changing to another design which is based on the same optical principle.

Summary

Presbyopes are increasing throughout Europe and the demand for presbyopic contact lens correction will, inevitably, continue to increase. There is an enormous untapped interest in contact lens wear among pres-

---

Key points

- The number of presbyopic patients requiring contact lens correction is increasing and is predicted to continue to do so over the next five years.
- In fitting the presbyope, the practitioner should have access to a number of different lens designs and be aware of alternative fitting approaches.
- The availability of single use disposable trial lenses allows ease of trial for both patients and practitioners.
- Lens power adjustments should not be based on measured visual acuity alone.
- Subjective visual performance assessment is most effectively achieved by experiencing lens wear in both the work and home environment.
- There is a significant untapped opportunity for contact lens correction of presbyopes.

---

byopes. Being aware of the different lens designs, fitting approaches and the associated advantages and disadvantages along with the patient's personality, occupation and previous lens wearing history helps in understanding which is the more appropriate starting point in meeting the patient's particular visual needs.

There are now more lens options than ever to offer our presbyopic patients and the lack of the 'perfect' contact lens solution for the presbyope should not discourage practitioners from fitting this ever-increasing patient base. New simultaneous designs with improved optical performance are now relatively easy to fit and the increasing availability of single-use diagnostic trial lenses allows effective trials to help eliminate failures prior to dispensing. If the initial lens powers selected fails to provide adequate visual performance, alternative fitting approaches such as enhanced and modified monovision can be explored. With experience, alternating lens designs can be added to the lens choice to offer patients bifocal correction if more exacting visual performance is required. In addition, the simplicity of monovision remains an effective solution for many presbyopes.

Question 8.1

If a +2.00 blur test results in the patient reporting that the image is clearest when the +2.00D lens is held in front of the left eye, then:

  A The patient is left eye dominant
  B No strong dominance is present
  C The patient is right eye dominant
  D The patient is left handed
  E The patient is right handed

Question 8.2

Which of the following is NOT an advantage of monovision?

  A Good near vision performance
  B Success rates at least equal to bifocal lens fitting
  C Easy to trial
  D Full stereopsis
  E Full choice of lens design and material type

Question 8.3

Which of the following statements regarding alternating bifocal lenses is FALSE?

  A Fused and solid designs are available
  B Are usually fitted steeper than flattest K
  C Visual quality is high with successful fits
  D Prism is used to control lens stability and position
  E Lower eyelid tone is important to enable adequate lens translation

Question 8.4

Which of the following statements is FALSE in relation to simultaneous vision lens fitting?

  A Lens centration is important
  B 0.25D adjustments can have a profound effect on visual performance
  C Over-refraction using a phoropter is preferred
  D Objective vision measurement alone is not a good predictor of success
  E Modified and enhanced monovision fitting techniques can be explored when necessary

Question 8.5

Back-surface aspheric soft lens designs are usually:

  A Centre-near type designs
  B Distance image bias in high luminance lighting levels
  C Distance image bias in low luminance lighting levels

  D Designed to correct greater than 1.50D of presbyopia
  E Near image bias in low luminance lighting levels

Question 8.6

Modified monovision fitting approach involves:

  A Reducing the add power during monovision fitting
  B Fitting one eye with a single-vision lens and the other with a bifocal
  C Ensuring both eyes are fitted with alternative centre-near designs
  D Fitting a translating lens design in one eye and a simultaneous lens design in the other
  E Altering distance or near power to enhance distance vision in one eye and near in the other

Question 8.7

The percentage of UK presbyopic patients over the age of 45 is:

  A 16 per cent
  B 31 per cent
  C 47 per cent
  D 28 per cent
  E 64 per cent

Question 8.8

Which of the following statements is TRUE about multi-zone concentric bifocal designs?

  A Allow distance and near vision by lens translation
  B Enhance near image contrast in high luminance lighting
  C Consist of two distance powered zones and one near
  D Minimize the dependency of lens function on pupil size
  E Enhance near image contrast in low luminance lighting levels

Question 8.9

When fitting alternating vision bifocals, the segment top position during primary gaze should be approximately:

  A Midway between lower pupil margin and inferior limbus
  B In line with the lower pupil margin
  C Bisecting the pupil horizontally
  D In line with the upper pupil margin
  E Midway between upper pupil margin and superior limbus

Question 8.10

Which of the following statements is FALSE about simultaneous vision correction?

  A Are available in both soft and rigid materials
  B Rely on the visual system to 'select' the clearer picture
  C Result in less reduction in stereopsis when compared to monovision
  D Result in the same subjective and objective visual performance as a spectacle lens correction
  E Lens adjustments can be made based on knowledge of ocular dominance

References

1 Papas, E., Young, G. and Hearn, K. (1990) Monovision versus soft diffractive bifocal contact lenses: a crossover study. *ICLC* **17**:181–186.

2 Back, A.P., Woods, R. and Holden, B.A. (1997) The comparative visual performance of monovision and various concentric bifocals. *Trans BCLA* 46–47.

3 Harris, M.G., Sheeny, J.E. and Gan, C.M. (1992) Vision and task performance with monovision and diffractive bifocal contact lenses. *Optom Vis Sci* **69:8** 609–614.

4 Molinary, J.F. (1998) A clinical comparison of subjective effectiveness of monovision, aperture-dependent and independent bifocal hydrogel lens fittings. *Trans BCLA* 58–59.

5 Saunders, B.D. (1989) The optical performance of bifocal contact lenses. *Trans BCLA* 71–74.

6 MacAlister, G.O. and Woods, C.A. (1991) Monovision versus RGP translating bifocals. *JBCLA* **14:4** 173–178.

7 Dutoit, R., Situ, P., Simpson, T. and Fonn, D. (2000) Results of one year clinical trial comparing monovision and bifocal contact lenses. *Optom Vis Sci* **77** S18.

8 Morgan, P. and Efron, N. (2000) Trends in UK contact lens problem-solving. *Optician* **219:5749** 22–23.

9 Edwards, K. (2000) Progressive power contact lens problem solving. *Optician* **219:5749** 16–20.

10 Woods, C., Ruston, D., Hough, T. and Efron, N. (1999) Clinical performance of an innovative back surface multifocal contact lens in correcting presbyopia. *CLAO Journal* **25:3** 176–181.

11 Plakitsi, A. and Charman, W.N. (1995) Comparison of the depths of focus with

the naked eye with three types of presbyopic contact lens correction. *JBCLA* **18:4** 119–125.

12 Meyler, J. and Veys, J. (1999) A new 'pupil-intelligent' lens for presbyopic correction. *Optician* **217:5687** 18–23.

13 Michaud, L., Tchang, J.P., Baril, C. and Gresset, J. (1995) New perspectives in monovision: a study comparing aspheric with disposable lenses. *ICLC* **22** 203–208.

14 Schor, C., Landsman, L. and Erickson, P. (1987) Ocular dominance and the interocular suppression of blur in monovision. *Am J Optom* **64** 723–730.

15 Erickson, P. (1998) Potential range of clear vision in monovision. *J Am Optom Assoc* **59:** 203–205.

16 Harris, M.G. (1993) Keep presbyopic contact lens wearers informed. *CL Spectrum* **9:** 50–53.

17 Benjamin, W.J. and Borish, I.M. (1994) Presbyopia and the influence of ageing on prescription of contact lenses. In: Rubin, M. and Guillon, M. eds. *Contact Lens Practice.* Chapman and Hall Medical 783–829.

18 Collins, M.J. and Bruce, A.S. (1994) Factors influencing performance with monovision. *JBCLA* **17:3** 91–96.

9
Contact lens aftercare

Introduction

It is generally accepted that many of the skills needed for contact lens practice have moved from fitting to aftercare as contact lens manufacturing technology, materials and design have advanced.

Currently available contact lenses provide the highest margin of safety since the introduction of the contact lens. It must be remembered, however, that contact lenses are medical devices that are primarily used to correct refractive errors.

Unlike spectacles, they are placed in direct contact with living anterior ocular tissue, and, as such, the potential for physiological changes exists. Experience and research, however, have shown that the incidence of serious complications is very low.

Despite this, the importance of contact lens aftercare cannot be over-emphasized, particularly given the high number of people ceasing to wear contact lenses (around 50 per cent in some studies). The main reasons cited for the high drop-out rates are discomfort (25 per cent) and dry eye (20 per cent).[1] Most of these drop-outs are avoidable, however, with regular comprehensive aftercare, improved communication between the practitioner and patient and adopting the use of higher performance lenses and/or care systems. The most successful aftercare often follows the old adage that 'prevention is better than cure', with the most effective way to manage complications being to avoid them.

It is often said that 'aftercare' begins before a contact lens is placed on the patient's eye. It is certainly true that the standards for successful continuing contact lens wear and care should be established at the first consultation. Communication is the key to establishing a good relationship between the practitioner and patient, so that the former can fully understand the needs and expectations of the patient to enable him or her to make the best professional recommendations for each individual. In turn, an informed patient will understand the importance of correct lens wear and care and the need for ongoing aftercare.

It is not sufficient, however, just to verbally communicate findings and instructions, as the need to keep meticulous records of all visits, findings, instructions and actions to be taken is of vital importance and is in the best interests of both the patient and practitioner. Guidelines for record keeping are provided by professional bodies, and the practitioner should be aware that comprehensive record keeping is often a statutory requirement.

Instrumentation

The basic instrumentation required for contact lens aftercare is the same that is needed to fit either soft or rigid contact lenses. The key instrument, the slit-lamp, has already been discussed in detail in Chapter 2. It should again be noted that a slit-lamp incorporating a graticule allows a more objective and accurate measurement of findings.

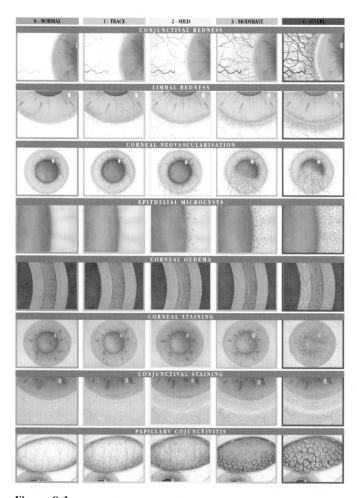

Figure 9.1
Efron Grading Scales.

When the measurement of a slit-lamp finding on a continuous scale cannot be carried out, a suitable grading scale should be adopted. Whatever grading scale is used, however, it is important that it is applied consistently and agreed and understood by all practitioners working in a practice. A written reference chart, or better still a photographic chart, such as that produced by the CCLRU or Efron (Figure 9.1), is the most effective. This can be supported further by the use of digital imaging systems.[2]

Clear and comprehensive record cards not only assist in the ongoing aftercare of a contact lens wearer, but are also required by law.

Techniques

Visit frequency and timings

The frequency of aftercare visits will vary for individual patients and lens types. A neophyte, in particular, will require closer monitoring in the early stages compared with an experienced contact lens wearer. Similarly, extended wear patients will require an appointment in the morning after the first night of sleeping in their lenses. After the initial programme of aftercare visits has been completed and the practitioner is happy with the lens performance and patient compliance, a six-monthly, or at least an annual, visit is usually sufficient for lenses worn on a daily wear basis.

It is also not sufficient only to offer ongoing aftercare, as practitioners have a professional duty to ensure it is provided. This can be achieved by using a patient reminder/tracking system. The use of computer-assisted systems is invaluable in this process, and a good practical tip is to make the next aftercare appointment before the patient leaves the practice and then call the patient a week or two before the appointment to check that he or she can still attend. The timing of the aftercare appointment is also important. For all lens types worn on a daily wear basis, patients should ideally be examined in the afternoon following several hours of contact lens wear. For those wearing lenses overnight, an early morning appointment as soon as possible after waking is best.

For all routine aftercare visits, patients should be instructed to attend the appointment wearing their contact lenses,

unless, of course, there is a specific reason not to, such as painful red eye. It is also helpful if patients bring their contact lens case, all the solutions used and their spectacles with them, as 'pictures' speak a thousand words!

Contact lens patients are notorious for believing that regular visits are unnecessary as long as their lenses are still comfortable and their vision is clear. Practitioners need to ensure patients understand the need for routine ongoing aftercare and that, although symptoms are warning signs, not all possible complications have symptoms, such as vascularization, staining and low-grade oedema. As with the contact lens screening examination, developing a routine for an aftercare examination ensures a full procedure is carried out efficiently and in a timely way. It is common to start with the patient discussion, before moving on to the examination with lenses *in situ*, followed by an investi-

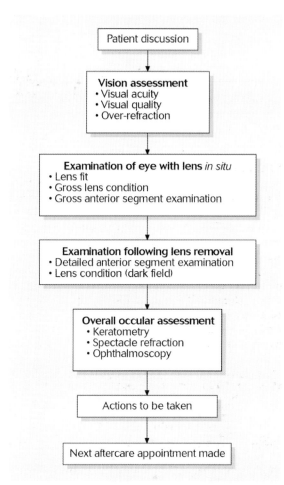

Figure 9.2
Suggested routine for an aftercare examination.

gation immediately after lens removal and, finally, a discussion of actions to be taken (Figure 9.2).

Patient discussion

Discussions about their history and symptoms with patients are a vital aspect of the aftercare examination. As with the pre-screening examination, a great deal of attention must be paid to the questioning technique. It is critical to ask for information in a way that encourages the patient to talk. Hence open, rather than closed, questions should be used. Reviewing lens care instructions is of particular importance, as this is an area in which compliance and/or misunderstanding is often poorest. Patients should be asked to demonstrate and describe their lens care routine, and practitioners should respond by praising where praise is due, hence reinforcing

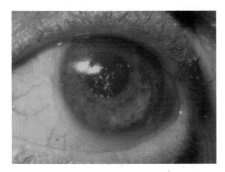

Figure 9.3
Jelly bumps seen with the lens in situ.

correct actions, in addition to correcting poor practice and highlighting areas of non-compliance.

The use of observation skills will also assist the practitioner in his or her assessment of patient compliance, such as the cleanliness of hands, length of fingernails, state of the lens case and how much solution is being used. Table 9.1 provides a guideline for the questions that need to be addressed with patients at an aftercare visit. In addition to open questions from the practitioner, it is important to encourage the patient to ask questions as the discussion progresses.

Examination (lenses *in situ*)

Vision assessment

Visual quality, in addition to visual acuity, should be assessed. The measurement of visual acuity (VA) is a legal requirement that must be undertaken and recorded before a physical examination of the eye is carried out. Visual acuity measurement is, however, a poor indicator of overall visual quality or patient satisfaction with the lenses' visual performance. Studies have indicated a poor correlation between VA and subjective visual quality [3], which can be objectively recorded using either a simple five-point scale or by using visual analogue scales.

Visual acuity should be measured and recorded monocularly and binocularly, and any over-refraction determined. The use of a retinoscope can be helpful in assessing both the quality of the reflex and the degree of over-refraction required. An assessment of the binocular vision status should also be carried out. This is of particular importance for higher prescriptions, in which the oculomotor balance can be very different from that with spectacles due to differences in prismatic effects.

Slit-lamp examination

With the lenses *in situ*, the slit-lamp can be utilzed to assess the lens fit and gross deposition.

Lens fit
For soft lenses, the corneal coverage, centration, edge alignment, primary gaze movement and the push-up test should be carried out. For rigid lenses, corneal coverage, centration, movement with blinks and corneal alignment should be assessed. Other observations, such as air bubbles or debris trapped under the lenses, should also be recorded. The wearers' blink rate and the completeness of the blink can also be assessed. With rigid lenses, in particular, the position of the upper lid should also be noted. Long-term rigid contact lens wear has been shown to be associated with increased ptosis, which can be monitored with ongoing aftercare and comparisons made with baseline measurements.

Lens condition
Only a gross assessment of the front-surface lens deposition can be made with the lenses *in situ* (Figure 9.3). A more satisfactory assessment of lens spoilation using dark-field illumination following lens removal is described later in this chapter. The measurement of the pre-lens tear film by non-invasive methods will also assist the practitioner in assessing the lens surface quality and the degree to which deposition is potentially interfering with maximum lens comfort.

Examination (after lens removal)

At this stage of the examination, contact lenses should be removed from the eyes and, ideally, temporarily stored in appropriate soaking solution in the patient's case. Allowing patients to remove at least one of

Wearing habits	How many days per week? How many hours per day? Do you even sleep in your contact lenses? How many nights per week?
Lens performance	How old are your lenses? How often do you replace your lenses? Do your experience any problems with your lenses? How is your vision? How do your lenses feel?
Handling	Tell me how you put your lenses in Tell me how you take your lenses out Probe hand washing procedure and frequency
Lens care	Do you care for your lenses? Demonstrate procedure Review cleaning/rinsing/disinfecting – procedure – frequency How often do you store your lenses when they are not being worn? Other solutions/tablets?
If problem	Are both eyes affected? When did you first notice the problem? Has the problem remained constant or varied? Is it worse at any particular time? (after insertion/after x hours/at the end of the day) Have you experienced the problem before? Does the problem persist after lens removal? Have you taken any treatment to date?
Spectacles	Do you have an up-to-date pair of spectacles?

Table 9.1
Questions to be addressed with contact lens wearers at an aftercare examination.

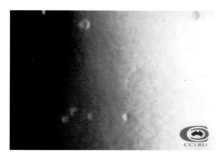

Figure 9.4
Microcysts as observed by retro-illumination.

their lenses will permit the practitioner to assess the wearer's techniques for lens removal, which is of more relevance to new wearers.

The aftercare routine outlined so far has been to assess the performance of the contact lenses themselves. The next stage is designed to reveal ocular changes induced by lens wear. Since a corneal change may be revealed by either an alteration in the optical characteristics of the eye or a change in its appearance, tests for both must be carried out. Hence, a slit-lamp examination is required to make an assessment of the anterior ocular tissues, and retinoscopy, subjective refraction and keratometry are used to assess the eyes' optical behaviour.

Slit-lamp examination
Anterior segment examination
It should be noted that signs of acute corneal oedema might fade quickly after lens removal, and so tests for its presence should be carried out first. For hard non gas-permeable lens wearers significant corneal oedema can result and it manifests itself as central corneal clouding (CCC), which can be viewed using the sclerotic scatter illumination technique with the slit-lamp, assisted by a darkened room. The CCC

should be graded according to the density (0 for not present to four for heavy), extent (the area covered in both horizontal and vertical meridians) and depth (epithelial or stromal).

For all soft lens wearers and modern rigid gas-permeable materials levels of oedema are significantly less than for non gas-permeable lenses and the clinical signs of oedema are more subtle. This can manifest as epithelial microcysts and stromal striae. It is easy to overlook epithelial microcysts, which can look like tear film debris and in small numbers are often asymptomatic. They are most effectively viewed using retro-illumination and appear as small, immobile inclusions exhibiting reversed illumination (Figure 9.4). Their appearance in small numbers is unremarkable, however, but a large number (>30) is indicative of corneal epithelial metabolic distress. With currently available high-performance lenses and materials, corneal oedema should not exceed 5 per cent during daily wear. As vertical striae appear at approximately 5 per cent to 6 per cent of oedema, they are an important observation at an aftercare visit and suggest that action is required.[4]

After examining for signs of corneal oedema, a full slit-lamp routine should be carried out to assess the anterior ocular adnexa in detail. Adverse effects, such as limbal vessel engorgement, conjunctival hyperaemia and corneal infiltrates (Figure 9.5), should all be noted and graded.

The use of fluorescein is imperative at every aftercare visit for both rigid and soft lens wearers. If any residual fluorescein remains in the eye after the examination, it should be rinsed out prior to a soft lens being inserted. In practice, as long as a minimal amount of fluorescein is inserted, most will have been excreted before the

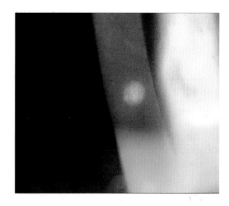

Figure 9.5
Corneal infiltrate with no overlying epithelial staining (courtesy of Joanne Boyd).

lenses are reinserted. The area covered and the extent and depth of epithelial staining should be graded. The pattern of staining, in particular, provides the practitioner with the greatest clue to the cause (Figure 9.6).

Lid eversion is also necessary at every aftercare visit to monitor for allergic reactions – particularly for signs of hyperaemia and the position (Figure 9.7), type, size and number of follicles and/or papillae. Lid margins should also be observed. Oedema of the lids resulting from contact lens wear may be due to thick, rough or poorly contoured edges, or indeed a poorly fitting lens. The meibomian glands should also be examined for patency and any signs of dysfunction. In conclusion, all observations should be graded, recorded and compared with baseline records, when available.

Lens condition
The slit-lamp can also be used to assess the lens condition *in vitro*, and using dark field illumination gives a far better indication of the nature and extent of lens spoilation, as shown in Figures 9.8(a) and 9.8(b). The

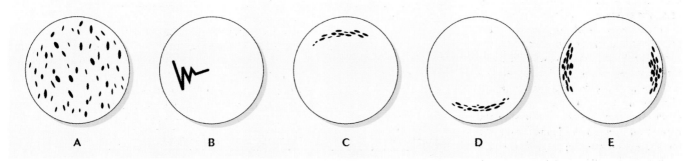

Figure 9.6
Likely causes of epithelial staining. A = toxic reaction, B = foreign body, C = hypoxic/mechanical, D = desiccation (soft), E = desiccation (rigid).

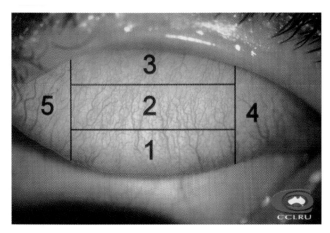

Figure 9.7
CCLRU system for recording position of lid redness and roughness.

lens should first be rubbed and rinsed with saline, then held with plastic coated tweezers and rinsed again to remove loosely attached debris. It should then be held in the slit-lamp beam, with light directed tangentially and the concave side pointing towards the eyepiece. The practitioner can then assess the spoilation of the lens under magnification against a dark background and grade the deposit in terms of its type, area and extent.

Keratometry
With rigid lenses in particular, it is useful to monitor corneal curvature for signs of steeping, flattering or distortion. Small-induced changes in K-readings are generally insignificant unless accompanied by other signs of corneal change. Of greater importance is any irregularity in the shape of the keratometer mire images, with distortion suggesting damage to the epithelium and likely to cause disturbance in vision.

Spectacle refraction
Retinoscopy
The quality of reflex should be carefully observed, and any areas of newly acquired irregular reflex characteristics noted. A central shadow, for example, can be indicative of a surface refractive effect rather than an opacity.

Subjective refraction
Spectacle blur and poor end-points in refraction are gradually becoming rarer as fewer patients continue to wear hard PMMA contact lenses. When encountered, however, these patients can often be difficult to manage at an aftercare visit,

particularly if they request a spectacle prescription for use on lens removal. The most effective medium and long-term management is to refit with rigid gas-permeable lenses to allow improved corneal physiology and a reduction in corneal distortion over time. For most patients, the most appropriate time for determining their spectacle prescription is immediately following lens removal.

It must always be remembered that reduced acuity in contact lens wearers might not be a result of either a refractive change or corneal distortion. As with routine examinations, the practitioner should always remain vigilant at an aftercare examination for the presence of any pathology.

Ophthalmoscopy
Every aftercare visit does not always necessitate ophthalmoscopy, although it should be carried out, or arrangement made for a full eye examination, at least annually (or sooner if suspicious signs or symptoms present). It can be useful to carry out

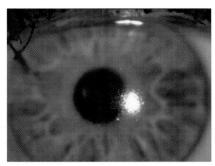

Figure 9.8(a)
Gross assessment of deposition with lens in situ (courtesy of Lyndon Jones).

ophthalmoscopy with the contact lenses *in situ*, particularly with high myopes or in the presence of gross corneal irregularity, as the lens greatly aids observation.

Interpretation of results

In deciding the course of action to be taken, the results from the tests, measurements, observations carried out in the aftercare examination and information provided by the patient have to be taken into consideration.

Contact lens problems may be the result of one or more of the following: toxic/allergic; mechanical/trauma; metabolic/hypoxic; and inflammatory/infection. During the course of the aftercare examination, the practitioner needs to evaluate signs and symptoms to address any actual or potential complications. With increased clinical experience, practitioners become more adept at resolving problems based on patients' reported symptoms and the assessment of observed signs. It is, of course, important to differentiate between a symptom and a sign. A symptom is when a patient complains of a physical problem, such as dryness, visual blur or pain, whereas a sign is the physical manifestation of a problem that is observed during the aftercare examination. Not all symptoms are associated with signs, however, and not all signs have symptoms. It is also important to differentiate between normal signs and the symptoms of contact lens wear, particularly those experienced during the adaptation period for new lens wear, such as lens awareness, and mild photophobia.

Table 9.2 summarizes the common signs and symptoms seen in routine contact lens practice and suggests actions

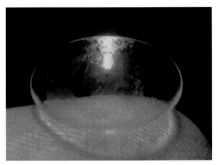

Figure 9.8(b)
Assessment of deposition in vitro using dark field illumination (courtesy of Lyndon Jones).

Symptoms	Signs/cause	Action
Discomfort on insertion or sudden onset	Foreign body	Remove lens, rinse and reinsert
	Damaged lens	Replace lens
	Decentred lens	Re-centre – if reoccurs check lens fit
	Conjunctival infection from chemical contamination	Remove lens, rinse and reinsert
	Excessive lens movement	Lens inside out – correct
	Corneal abrasion	Cease lens wear for 24 hours and reinsert. If symptoms reoccur, seek immediate advice
Discomfort after a period of wear	Lens deposition	Replace lens
	Lens dehydration	Wetting drops, increase lens replacement frequency, review blink action
	Three and nine o'clock staining	Improve centration, reduce edge clearance, refit with soft
	Poor lens wetting	Replace lens
	Trapped debris under lens	Remove lens, rinse and reinsert
	Toxic reaction to solution	Change care system
	Contact lens-associated papillary conjunctivitis/CLPC	Increase lens replacement frequency and/or change care system
Discomfort after lens removal	Oedema due to tight lens	Change lens fit, refit with higher oxygen permeable lens
	Corneal abrasion	Remove lens, resolve cause
	Corneal inflammation	Remove lens until signs resolve
	Corneal infection (microbial keratitis)	Seek immediate ophthalmological advice
Discomfort periodically	Lens surface drying	Blinking exercises if due to incomplete blink
	Environmental factors (smoke or low humidity)	Avoid these environments
Blurred vision constant	Lenses switched eyes	Re-switch back
	Incorrect prescription	Refract and provide new prescription
	Residual astigmatism	Refit with RGP or soft toric
	Distorted lens	Replace lens
Blurred vision fluctuation with blink		
– better post-blink	Lens deposits	Replace lens
– worse post-blink	Excessive lens movement/loose lens fit	Refit
	Lens inside out	Correct
Blurred vision over time Worse towards end of day	Corneal oedema	Refit with higher oxygen permeable lens
	Lens surface drying	Clean and/or replace lens
	Lens deposits	Replace lens
Fluctuating vision from day to day	Contact lens-associated papillary conjunctivitis/CLPC	Increase lens replacement frequency
	Environmental factors (smoke and low humidity)	Avoid cause
Spectacle blur after lens removal	Distorted cornea	Refit all PMMA wearers with RGP lenses
Flare (reflections, ghost images, diplopia)		Improve rigid lens fit
	Decentred lens	Refit/improve centration
	BOZD or FOZD too small	Refit, larger BOZD and/or FOZD
	Residual astigmatism	Refit with RGP or soft toric
	Severe deposition	Replace lens
None	Corneal staining	Remove lens, resolve cause
	Vascularization	Refit with higher oxygen permeable lens
	Low to moderate oedema	Refit with higher oxygen permeable lens

Table 9.2
Common symptoms, signs, causes and actions to be taken if encountered at an aftercare examination.

for each of the conditions. The differential diagnosis and management of contact-lens related changes can be reviewed further from the literature.[5,6]

Serious complications are rare, however accurate diagnosis and management are critical if they present in practice. The key differences between microbial keratitis and sterile keratitis (CLPU: contact lens peripheral ulcer) are shown in Table 9.3. The former requires urgent referral for immediate ophthalmological investigation whereas the latter can often be managed by the contact lens practitioner.

Recommendations to wearers

The advice given to patients must be based on the condition of the patients' eyes and lenses. Recommendations should be clear, and the use of jargon avoided, while verbal instructions should be backed up by written instructions. The reason for, and benefits of, particular recommendations and actions should always be explained. Patients are sometimes unwilling to take the advice given, especially if they are unaware of any symptoms. They should be warned of the possible outcome if the advice is ignored and, in the case of potentially serious consequences, it may be advisable to suggest that another opinion be sought. A brief summary of the advice given should always be noted on the patient record card for both future reference and legal purposes.

The necessity of continued regular aftercare visits must be stressed and re-stressed to all contact lens wearers, new or established. It is always beneficial, especially for new wearers, to make the next appointment at the end of the current visit. In addition to scheduled routine aftercare appointments, patients must be instructed to contact the practice if any problems or uncertainty about their lens wear occurs. Figure 9.9 shows a decision tree that a contact lens wearer should follow if experiencing problems.

Key points

- Comprehensive aftercare is an essential part of contact lens practice, irrespective of the patients' symptoms.
- Practitioners should develop a full aftercare routine to ensure all necessary assessments are carried out and recorded appropriately.
- Aftercare should incorporate both objective and subjective assessments of the lens performance and effect.
- Attention should also be paid to ocular function and structures not directly in contact with the lens.

Summary

The aim of aftercare is to determine an individual's response to contact lens wear, confirm compliance with instructions and detect and prevent potential problems. This involves assessing the integrity of the eye before and after wearing contact lenses and

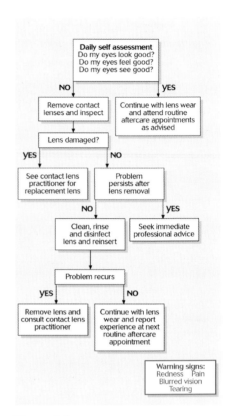

Figure 9.9
Daily decision tree for a contact lens wearer.

trying to minimize any induced ocular changes. Paying close attention to comprehensive aftercare enables practitioners to maintain close links with their patients, to the mutual benefit of both practitioners and patients.

Question 9.1
Which lens fitting will subsequently require more frequent initial and ongoing aftercare?
A   Neophyte daily wear new fit
B   Existing daily wear refit to alternative daily wear lens
C   Neophyte extended wear new fit
D   Existing extended wear refit to daily wear modality
E   Existing extended wear refit to alternative extended wear lens

Question 9.2
Which of the following clinical observations is more likely to result in patient symptoms?
A   Vascularization
B   Microcysts
C   Low-grade CLPC
D   Infiltrate (no overlying epithelial staining)

	Presumed microbial	Presumed sterile
Symptoms and signs	Central lesions	Peripheral lesions
	Lesions >1mm diameter	Lesions <1mm diameter >1mm within the limbal zone
	Epithelial defect	Intact epithelium (early) or late epithelial defect
	Severe pain	Mild pain
	Progressive pain	Non-progressive pain
	Severe corneal suppuration	Mild corneal suppuration
	Progressive corneal suppuration	Non-progressive suppuration
	Uveitis	No uveitis

Table 9.3
Differential diagnosis of infected and sterile keratitis.

E   Diffuse epithelial staining resulting from toxic reaction

Question 9.3
Which aspects of vision assessment would not be carried out routinely during contact lens aftercare?
   A   Visual acuity
   B   Stereopsis
   C   Oculomotor balance
   D   Subjective visual quality
   E   Quality of retinoscopy reflex

Question 9.4
Acute and/or chronic corneal oedema resulting from soft lens wear will not result in which of the following clinical signs?
   A   Microcysts
   B   Central corneal clouding
   C   Vertical striae
   D   Vascularization
   E   Epithelial staining

Question 9.5
Which of the following is imperative at every aftercare visit?
   A   Use of fluorescein during slit-lamp examination
   B   Keratometry measurements
   C   Ophthalmoscopy
   D   Spectacle refraction
   E   Lid eversion

Question 9.6
Which of the following signs/symptoms is more typical of a sterile keratitis?
   A   Central lesion
   B   Lesion >1 mm
   C   Uveitis
   D   Progressive clinical signs
   E   Mild pain

Question 9.7
Which of the following statements concerning aftercare appointments is true?
   A   Patients should decide the frequency of visit
   B   Aftercares are only needed whenever a patient is suffering any symptoms of discomfort
   C   The patient should always attend wearing their current contact lenses except in unusual circumstances
   D   Vision is assessed during routine eye examinations so is not a consideration at an aftercare appointment
   E   Reminders to patients to attend for aftercare appointments have proven useless

Question 9.8
Which of the following is most likely to lead to an inferior corneal 'smile' stain?
   A   Toxic response
   B   Foreign body beneath the upper lid
   C   Hypoxic response
   D   Desiccation with soft lens wear
   E   Desiccation with RGP lens wear

Question 9.9
Which of the following statements concerning visual compromise reported at an aftercare appointment is true?
   A   Deposits would lead to an improved acuity post-blink
   B   Deposits would lead to a reduced acuity post-blink
   C   A loose fitting lens would give an improved acuity post-blink
   D   A lens that was inside out would give an improved post-blink acuity
   E   Corneal oedema would give an improved post-blink acuity

Question 9.10
Which of the following would typically cause a gradual worsening of acuity as the day progresses?
   A   Loose-fitting lens
   B   Flare
   C   Foreign body
   D   Corneal oedema
   E   Inappropriate refractive correction

References

1   Weed, K. H., Fonn, D. and Potuin, R. (1993) Discontinuation of contact lens wear. *Optom Vis Sci* **70:12** 140.
2   Meyler, J. and Burnett-Hodd, N. (1998) The use of digital image capture in contact lens practice. *Contact Lens and Anterior Eye* **21S**: s3–s11.
3   Davies, I. P., Inglis, A. and Davies, G. (1992) Correlation between visual acuity and visual quality in contact lens practice. *JBCLA* **15:4** 155–157.
4   Efron, N. (1991) Understanding oxygen: Dk/L, EOP, oxygen. *JBCLA* **14:2** 65–69.
5   Stapleton, F, Dart, J. (1995) Management of contact lens-related disease. *Optician* **210:5530** 21–26.
6   Covey, M. and Munro, F. (1999) Differential diagnosis in contact lens aftercare. *Optician* **217: 5691** 24–32.
7   Efron, N. (1999) *Contact Lens Complications.* Butterworth-Heinemann.
8   Jones, L. W. and Jones, D. A. (2000) *Common Contact Lens Complications.* Butterworth-Heinemann.
9   Bruce, A. S. and Brennan, N. A. (1990) Corneal pathophysiology with contact lens wear. *Surv Ophthalmol* **35:1** 25–58.

10
Contact lens care systems

Introduction

A wide range of care products are available today and the specific lens care system prescribed will depend on the lens type and individual patient factors. This chapter aims to provide a general overview of the principles of lens care and solution properties. It will not deal with specific details of brands, but comprehensive reviews are available from the literature.[1,2]

During wear, contact lenses become contaminated by tear components such as proteins and lipids, tear debris such as desquamated epithelial cells or environmental pollutants and, in some cases, eye make-up. Contamination is also possible during handling and storage. The purpose of a lens care system is to combat this contamination, keep deposits to a minimum and maintain lens safety, comfort and vision.

Care system components

Care systems range from one bottle of multifunction solution to a number of bottles of various solutions with different functions. Some care systems require multiple steps to

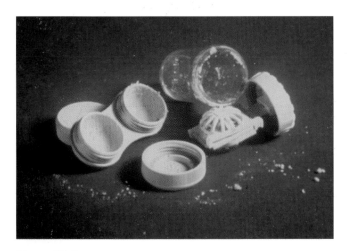

Figure 10.1
Lens cases: a significant source of contamination.

be carried out while others have approval to eliminate the 'rub' step. The basic steps are defined as follows:

Cleaning
This can be defined as the removal of surface deposits and other debris, usually achieved by rubbing the lens in the palm of the hand with a finger. A mechanical 'clean' can be achieved by rubbing the lens with sterile saline, but deposit removal will be facilitated by using solutions that are formulated to contain a surfactant cleaner (e.g. Poloxamer 407, tyloxapol) or other cleaning agent (e.g. citrate).

Other dedicated lens cleaners incorporate chemicals such as isopropyl alcohol or contain microscopic particles designed to be slightly abrasive. Not all surfactants act in the same way and some are more efficient than others at removing different substances from the lens surface. This is an important fact in problem-solving.

In addition to removing debris from the lens, the cleaning action removes bacteria from the surface and as such is an essential element in the disinfection process. While the exact amount of bacteria removed during the cleaning process is in some doubt, there is a consensus that there is a

1 to 4 log unit reduction. Cleaning is particularly important in the removal of *Acanthamoeba* cysts and trophozoites from the surfaces of hard and soft contact lenses.

Rinsing
Rinsing a contact lens is another integral part of the cleaning and disinfection process. Cleaning and rinsing together remove over 99 per cent of micro-organisms from the lens. Rinsing also removes loosely bound debris from the surface and any remaining dedicated cleaning solution, which could otherwise lead to discomfort on lens insertion.

Disinfection
This is defined as the destruction of micro-organisms, but not necessarily bacterial spores. Disinfection is thus a critical step in the care of both soft and hard contact lenses. Failure to disinfect has been shown to be a significant contributory factor in the aetiology of microbial keratitis. The International Organisation for Standardization (ISO) has been active in developing standards for the testing and classifying of contact lens products.[4] The current standard – ISO 14729 – sets primary and secondary standards for disinfection based on the selected test organisms which consist of three bacteria and two fungi as shown in Table 10.1. *Acanthamoeba* is not included in this standard at this time.

A disinfecting solution must also maintain the lens in a microbe-free condition when in storage and maintain lens hydration. These factors are important when considering the choice of system for trial lens disinfection. However, with the recent concerns regarding the theoretical risk of vCJD transmission by contact lenses, the use of sodium hypochlorite 2% for prion inactivation, has been recommended for rigid contact lens decontamination. The ideal procedure for non single-patient use soft lens disinfection has yet to be recommended.

Test organisms	Log reduction required at recommended disinfection time to pass stand-alone test	Log reduction required to pass regimen test
Bacteria: *Staphylococcus aureus* *Pseudomonas aeruginosa* *Serratia marcescens*	3.0 (99.9%)	Total combined log reduction at least 5.0 and 1.0 log reduction for any bacterium
Fungi: *Candida albicans* *Fusarium solani*	1.0 (90%)	No growth

Table 10.1
Standard for testing and clarifying contact lens care products (ISO 14729)[4].

Sterilization

Sterilization is defined as the total removal of all living micro-organisms, including spores. It is a standard manufacturing procedure that all soft contact lenses be sterilized before dispatch. Sterilization is most commonly achieved in an autoclave, where the product is sterilized at a particular heat for a given time, typically 115–118°C for 30 minutes.

Wetting

Wetting solutions are predominantly used in hard contact lens practice. They are typically placed on the lens before insertion. They have three principal uses:
• Minimizing initial discomfort upon lens insertion by acting as a lubricant between the lens and the cornea.
• Encouraging even distribution of tears over the lens on insertion.
• Acting as a buffer between the lens and the finger on insertion to reduce contamination.

The effect of the wetting solution is an immediate one, which dissipates after around 15 minutes.

Protein removal

Proteins from the tear film enter the matrix of a soft lens and become loosely attached to the surface of both hard and soft lenses within minutes of lens insertion. With time these proteins may become more aggressively bound to the lens and become denatured. Denatured protein leads to reduction in lens comfort, vision and overall satisfaction and can also lead to atopic reactions such as contact lens-induced papillary conjunctivitis and red-eye reactions.

Protein-removing tablets contain enzymes, which break down the bonds between protein molecules, enabling them to be rinsed away from the lens. More modern enzyme formulations, such as subtilisin A, result in fewer atopic reactions than protein remover tablets containing papain. Liquid formulations are also available which contain pancreatin as the active ingredient. It is important to note that all these treatments are only effective on active proteins. Once the protein becomes denatured, then its chemical composition changes and the enzyme can no longer break the molecule down. Thus if protein removal treatment is to be carried out, it must be done on a regular basis. With the advent of disposable and frequent replacement lenses, the need for protein-removing tablets has declined. In addition the formulations of 'second-generation' multi-purpose solutions have altered to include protein removing properties.

Solution properties

All lens care products which come into contact with the eye, either directly or indirectly, need to be chemically and physically balanced to achieve patient comfort and maintain ocular health. It is important to be familiar with the general properties of a solution, to enable alternative products to be recommended if a patient is experiencing a particular problem. The properties and effectiveness of care products can change with time and for this reason all solutions should be used before the expiry date. The general properties that require consideration include:
• *Tonicity* – the average osmolarity of the human tear film is around 320 mmol/kg with a range for 300–350 mmol/kg. This equates to a concentration of 0.9 per cent sodium chloride solution. Ideally, contact lens solutions should have a similar tonicity to the tear film to avoid discomfort when lenses with residual solution are placed on the eye. As solution tonicity increases, the comfort will decrease and conjunctival hyperaemia increase (Figure 10.2).[6] While changes in solution tonicity can cause discomfort and hyperaemia, this is not always accompanied by corneal staining and therefore discomfort and hyperaemia are effective 'early warning signals' preceding corneal damage.
• *pH* – this is the hydrogen ion concentration or acid/alkaline balance of the solution, and for comfort should be in the range 6.6 to 7.8 pH, and as close as possible to the average pH of human tears (7.45 ± 0.16). It should be noted that tear pH is not a static value and like that of other body fluids shows diurnal variation. The tear pH following prolonged eye closure will change.

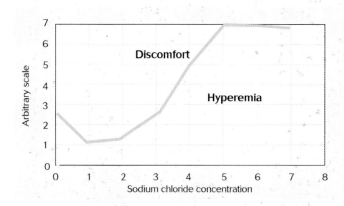

Figure 10.2
Effects of osmolarity on conjunctival hyperaemia and subjective comfort.

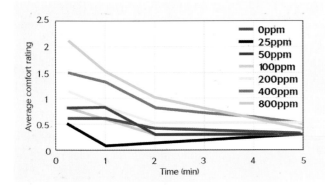

Figure 10.3(a)
Effect of residual hydrogen peroxide concentration on comfort[9].

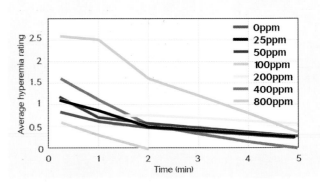

Figure 10.3(b)
Effect of residual hydrogen peroxide concentration on hyperaemia.[9]

The eye contains buffering agents, which are able to return the tear film to a normal pH if solutions beyond the normal range are inserted. However, the transient discomfort of this means that solutions should be as close as possible to the eyes' neutral pH. Differences do exist in the pH of solutions, for example between different aerosol salines and preserved salines, which can lead to discomfort in some patients. Buffered saline solution should lead to minimum discomfort.[7] Two commonly used buffers in contact lens solutions are borate and phosphate.

• *Viscosity* – viscosity agents can be incorporated to control the 'thickness' of the solution. The most commonly used viscosity-increasing agent is methylcellulose. This can be added to a wetting solution to increase contact time of the wetting agent to the lens, or be added to artificial tears to increase contact time of the formulation with the eye. The viscosity of surfactant cleaners can also be increased with a view to increasing contact time.

• *Disinfection agents* – once any contact lens solution has been opened, it is susceptible to microbial contamination. For this reason, all solutions other than single-use presentations or aerosols have to be preserved. The function of the preservative is to kill invading microbes. The chemicals used to preserve passively a contact lens solution may also be used to kill microbes in a disinfection solution.

Most disinfecting agents work by breaking

	Hydrogen peroxide two-step	Hydrogen peroxide one-step	Chlorine
Examples	Oxysept 1 and 2 (Allergan) 10:10 (Ciba Vision) Two-step peroxide (Sauflon)	Oxysept 1 step (Allergan) AOSept (Ciba Vision) EasySept (Bausch & Lomb)	Aerotab (Sauflon)
Principle	3% hydrogen peroxide used to disinfect the lens Minimum 10 minute neutralization step necessary before insertion into the eye	3% hydrogen peroxide used to disinfect the lens Delayed release neutralizing tablet or catalyst disc added at disinfecting stage	Chlorine-releasing tablet dissolved in unpreserved saline Chlorine acts to disinfect the lens
Advantages	Very efficient disinfection	More convenient than two-step system	Easy to use Economical
Disadvantages	Multiple steps Forgetting to neutralize will result in peroxide burn Possible parameter changes *	Possible film on some lenses Forgetting the tablet or an old disc will result in peroxide burn	Clean lens and case essential for effective disinfection Fogetting the tablet results in no disinfection
Full procedure	Soft contact lens cleaner Rinse Hydrogen peroxide (from 10 minutes to overnight) Neutralize Insert	Soft contact lens cleaner Rinse Hydrogen peroxide plus neutralizing tablet or catalyst disc (store overnight) Rinse Insert	Soft contact lens cleaner Rinse Unpreserved saline plus chlorine tablet (store overnight) Rinse Insert

* parameter changes can be resolved by a longer neutralization period

Table 10.2(a)
Types of oxidative or 'preservative free' care systems.

	Traditional	**High molecular weight**
Anti-microbial agent	Thiomersal Chlorhexidine	Polyhexanide Polyquad (Polydronium chloride)
Examples	No longer available Previous examples included Hydrocare PrymeCare OptimEyes	Complete Comfort Plus (Allergan) ReNu MultiPlus (Bausch & Lomb) All in One (Sauflon) Opti-free Express (Alcon) Solo-Care (Ciba Vision)
Principles	Anti-microbial agent is toxic to organisms resulting in disinfection during the storage period	Anti-microbial agent is toxic to organisms resulting in disinfection during the storage period
Advantages	Very easy to use Economical Ongoing disinfection	Very easy to use Economical Ongoing disinfection
Disadvantages	Ocular sensitivity and toxic reactions are common	Toxic reations may occur but are less common
Full procedure	Soft contact lens cleaner Rinse Soak for recommended disinfection cycle (minimum four hours) Rinse Insert	Clean Rinse Soak for recommended disinfection cycle (minimum four hours) Rinse Insert

Table 10.2(b)
Types of chemical or preservative-based disinfecting systems.

down the cell wall of the bacteria. Unfortunately, any compound which can break down bacterial cell walls is also able to break down epithelial cell walls and denature protein. In formulating a disinfection or preservative solution, a balance must be struck between a formulation strong enough to kill bacteria, yet mild enough not to become toxic to the eye or to cause irreversible changes to protein films on lenses.

An early attempt to achieve the balance

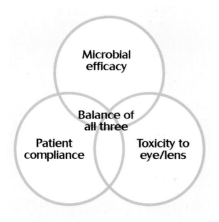

Figure 10.4
The balance that needs to be achieved for a successful care system.

was to use solutions such as chlorhexidine and thiomersal at very low concentrations. This strategy is successful from a passive preservative standpoint, but the solutions are not sufficiently bactericidal for use as a disinfectant without the incidence of atopic and toxic reactions increasing. With solutions such as this, the importance of the cleaning and rinsing steps was elevated.

Consequently solution manufacturers have moved towards the use of chemicals such as polyhexanide or polyquad (Polydronium chloride) as the principal disinfecting agent in so called 'multi-purpose solutions' (MPS). These lens care products are formulated to clean, rinse and disinfect soft contact lenses and their use is now well established. Although from the same family as chlorhexidine, these chemicals are less toxic to the eye than the older preservatives due to their larger molecular size preventing penetration of the preservative into the matrix of the hydrogel lens. In addition, each molecule causes proportionally more damage than traditional preservatives allowing lower concentrations to be formulated. This effectively reduces the potential for toxicity or sensitivity reactions,[8] although atopic reactions may still occur.

Most MPS solutions have a surfactant element built into the formulation. This surfactant may either act as a traditional surfactant cleaner or via the release of citrate which is thought to clean primarily by helping to solvate positively charged protein by ionic displacement. These products do vary in their preservative concentration as well as surfactant type and buffering agent, which may affect performance.[2] More recently, this first generation of MPS has been supplemented by new formulations with additional anti-microbial agents, cleaners, sequestering agents and wetting agents to improve efficacy and lens comfort.

Hydrogen peroxide is a very effective bactericidal agent but is also toxic to the eye, causing discomfort and conjunctival hyperaemia in concentrations over 100 ppm (Figure 10.3)[9]. In developing strategies to overcome this, solution manufacturers have relied on the relative ease with which hydrogen peroxide can be broken down into water and oxygen: $H_2O_2 <-> H_2O + O_2$.

To overcome the toxicity, solution systems have been developed where the lens is placed first in hydrogen peroxide and after an appropriate period of time (usually four hours to overnight soak) a catalyst is added which breaks down the peroxide. After a minimum of 10 minutes the lens can be placed on the eye without discomfort. Systems such as this add a third element into the efficacy/toxicity balance, which needs to be considered – that of ease of use. In addition, two-step hydrogen peroxide systems also change the parameters of lenses which are pH-sensitive. When ionic soft lenses are placed in hydrogen peroxide solutions their back optic radius and total diameter significantly decreases and the lens edge may appear 'fluted' and distorted. This change is reversible once the lens is neutralized, but it may take around 60 minutes for the lens to return to its original parameters. If a lens is placed in the eye after 20 minutes neutralization, around 20 per cent of patients will report discomfort on insertion and the lens will take up to one hour to show its correct fitting characteristics.[10]

In general, as discussed later, the easier a solution system is to use, the more likely the patient is to comply. The complexity of the early peroxide systems was not appreciated by many patients, but as systems have become easier to use, for example with the advent of 'one-step' peroxide solutions, then the relative microbial efficacy of the solution reduces as lenses are subjected to a lower exposure time to hydrogen peroxide. Such one-step systems can employ a platinum disc or a catalase tablet which when introduced together with the 3 per cent hydrogen peroxide initiate neutralization. When used in this way, one-step systems offer no on-going disinfection for intermittent users or for lenses in prolonged storage, which increases the potential for regrowth of bacteria and fungi.

The ideal care system must then have a balance of microbial efficacy, toxicity to the eye and ease of use/compliance (Figure 10.4). Tables 10.2(a) and 10.2 (b) show the basic types of care systems used in soft lens disinfection.

Although efficacy of disinfecting systems may vary, one study has shown no statistically significant difference in the expected risk of *Acanthamoeba* infection between contact lens wearers using hydrogen peroxide and multi-purpose solutions for disinfection of their lenses. Furthermore, no association was found with any particular FDA lens material type and risk of infection for hydrogen peroxide or multi-purpose solutions.[11]

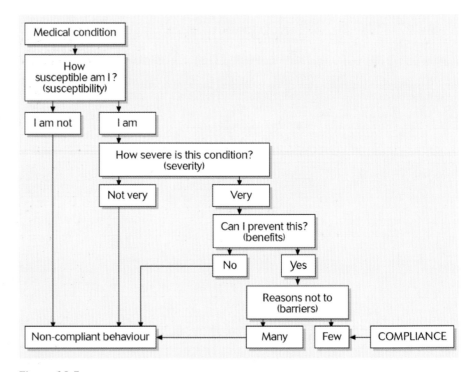

Figure 10.5
The human belief model by Becker and Maiman, cited by Sokol.[13]

Compounding factors

Handwashing
Patients should always be encouraged to wash their hands before handling lenses. For contact lens wearers, a thorough hand wash with soap and water is sufficient. Non-perfumed anti-bacterial liquid soap dispensers are preferable to bars of soap, which can become contaminated more easily. All soap must be thoroughly rinsed off the hands before the lenses are handled to avoid contamination. Hands should be dried on a clean lint-free towel. It is both comforting and of educational benefit for the patient to see practitioners wash their hands in the consulting room before handling lenses.

Case hygiene
As well as keeping the contact lens and the hands clean, it is important to keep the lens case clean. Lens cases have been shown to be a significant source of bacterial contamination. This contamination is made worse as bacteria adhering to the contact lens case become coated in a biofilm, which reduces the efficacy of care products. In

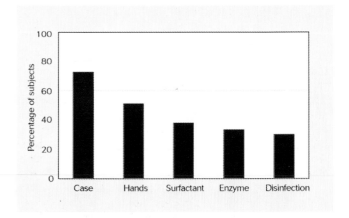

Figure 10.6
Incidence of non-compliant behaviour in a student population.[14]

Problem	Possible causes	Recommendations
Patient symptoms Poor vision		Increase lens replacement frequency
	Build-up of protein	Ensure MPS has protein removing properties. Change or introduce surfactant. Introduce protein treatment if necessary
	Lipid film	Introduce or change surfactant cleaner Try alternative lens material i.e. Group II to IV
Poor comfort on insertion	Residual peroxide on lens	Increase time in neutralizer. Use different peroxide solution
	Residual solution on lens	Rinse before insertion
	pH or tonicity imbalance with tear film	Rinse with isotonic buffered saline before insertion Change solution
	Ionic lens in overnight peroxide	Shorter peroxide exposure/longer neutralization Change to non-peroxide system
Poor comfort	Non-wetted lens (RGP)	Surfactant clean and rewet with wetting solution Change surfactant cleaner. Change wetting agent. Ensure lens has not been over-polished
	Atopic or toxic response	Change disinfecting solution to different action (alternative MPS with different preservative/concentration). Change to peroxide lens care system. Increase lens replacement frequency
Patient signs Increase in conjunctival hyperaemia	Atopic or toxic response	Increase lens replacement frequency Change disinfecting solution to different action (alternative MPS with different preservative/concentration). Change to peroxide lens care system
	pH or tonicity imbalance	Rinse with buffered isotonic saline before insertion. Change to alternative solutions with different buffer/pH
Increase in tarsal palpebral hyperaemia and/or papillae	Atopic or toxic solution reaction	Change disinfection solution to different action
Diffuse corneal staining	Atopic or toxic response	Change disinfection solution to different action Reduce concentration or type of protein remover tablet Ensure Px not using RGP solution with soft lenses
Lens deposits Protein	Old lens	Replace lens or increase replacement frequency
	Protein film	Ensure MPS has protein-removing properties. Introduce separate protein-removing cleaner
Lipid	Tear film quality	Introduce or change surfactant cleaner
Make-up	Make-up on lens	Introduce or change surfactant

Table 10.3
Systematic approach to problem-solving.

studies, more than 50 per cent of contact lens cases have been found to be contaminated with bacteria and 4 per cent with amoeboid species. On lens insertion, contact lens cases must be emptied of solution, rinsed with fresh disinfecting solution and left to air dry on a daily basis. A dry case is important as microbes cannot multiply in dry conditions.

Cases should also be replaced on a regular basis, at least every three months. Ideally, for frequent replacement lens wearers the new lens case should coincide with lens replacement. Some practitioners might also advise a weekly mechanical clean using a cotton bud moistened with contact lens cleaner. The case should then be rinsed with disinfecting solution and left to air dry. This mechanical scrub disrupts the biofilm.

Tap water
Since UK tap water has been implicated as a major source of *Acanthamoeba*, it should never come into contact with either the lens or lens case. Rigid gas-permeable (RGP) lens wearers may also be susceptible to contact lens related *Acanthamoeba*[11] infection and therefore caution should also prevail. Minimal advice to the RGP wearing patient should be to avoid tap water for rinsing their lenses immediately prior to lens insertion.

Compliance
Perhaps one of the most critical aspects in contact lens care is patient compliance – in other words how well the patient follows the instructions required for safe contact lens wear. Patient compliance is an issue in both contact lens wear and in general medicine and excellent reviews are available in the literature.[12,13]

The human belief model[14] can be illustrated by a flowchart used by a patient in deciding if they are going to be compliant with a procedure (Figure 10.5). The model shows that there are far more opportunities for a patient not to comply with a procedure than to follow it, particularly if the consequences of not following the procedure are felt to be unlikely to occur.

While it is generally accepted that most patients are non-compliant, it is equally well accepted that most believe that they are. The best way to find out if a patient is being compliant is to ask open questions about their care regime and ask the patient to demonstrate what they do. The importance of open questioning has been stressed throughout this book. Asking 'do you look after your lenses correctly?' is unlikely to produce a negative response, while 'show me what you do with your lenses when you remove them' provides more illuminating information.

Many studies have been carried out on different aspects of compliance. The studies support the human belief model in that a patient must understand that there is a real benefit to following instructions before they do so. This can be reinforced verbally – patients respond well to the approval of practitioners when they carry out an instruction or activity correctly. This reinforcement must be communicated throughout the aftercare procedure. Practitioners must also be aware of the best ways of explaining the consequences of non-compliance. Patients are less likely to respond to something that will 'stop you getting an infection', an unlikely event to them, than they are to something that will 'scratch the eyes', a phraseology that they can associate with and wish to avoid occurring.

Studies have shown that patients are far more likely to carry out procedures that affect comfort than safety. Figure 10.6 shows the results of a study carried out among students in London showing the incidence of non-compliant behaviour.[15] Nearly 30 per cent of patients failed to disinfect their soft lenses on removal.

Profile of non-compliant patient

It is possible to develop a profile of the patients who are most likely not to comply with instructions. Compliance decreases with younger patients, those who have been wearing lenses for a longer period of time, existing contact lens patients who are refitted, patients who wear lenses for long periods of time, and patients fitted for cosmetic rather than therapeutic reasons. It also decreases as care systems become more complex. However, patient non-compliance can be improved through practitioner re-instruction.

Problem-solving

Table 10.3 is a guide to some of the common problems that can be resolved by changes or modifications to care systems. The approach to problem-solving is the one advocated throughout this book – isolate the cause of the problem and then change the component in the lens/care system which affects that element.

Key points

- Any contact lens, whether soft or rigid, must be cleaned and disinfected following removal from the eye before it can be re-used.
- The solution selection for an individual patient is based on lens type, replacement schedule, wearing modality and patient profile.
- Careful patient instruction on correct cleaning and disinfecting procedures along with continual assessment during aftercare is the key to good patient compliance.
- Practise good hygiene in front of patients. Ask them to demonstrate their exact solution routine at aftercare visits.
- Be familiar with general properties of a solution to enable alternative products to be recommended if a patient is experiencing a particular problem.

Summary

Contact lens solutions play a critical part in the overall success of contact lens wear. An understanding of their properties and performance helps practitioners both to select an appropriate system for individual patients and resolve any problems that may arise during lens wear.

Question 10.1

Which of the following ocular conditions would not be due to a solution reaction?

A Diffuse corneal staining
B Corneal ulceration
C Conjunctival staining
D Conjunctival hyperaemia
E Tarsal palpebral hyperaemia and follicles

Question 10.2

Which of the following statements regarding 3% hydrogen peroxide is false?

A Hydrogen peroxide is an effective bactericidal agent
B Hydrogen peroxide can be broken down into oxygen and water
C Hydrogen peroxide can cause changes to soft lens parameters
D Hydrogen peroxide does not need neutralizing before lens insertion
E Hydrogen peroxide systems are generally free from preservatives

Question 10.3

Poor comfort on lens insertion could not be due to?

A Residual peroxide on lens
B Non-wetted lens
C Tonicity imbalance with tear film
D Residual cleaning solution on lens
E Build up of active protein

Question 10.4

Which of the following should not be considered when selecting an appropriate solution system for an individual patient?

A Lens type
B Replacement schedule
C Patient profile
D Wearing modality
E Lens power

Question 10.5

Soft contact lens sterilization can be achieved by:

A Soaking in disinfection solution alone
B Cleaning step prior to soaking in disinfection solution
C Heat to 80°C for 20 minutes
D Heat to 118°C for 30 minutes
E Soaking in 3 per cent hydrogen peroxide

Question 10.6

Which of the following statements is false?

A Denatured protein can lead to reduced lens comfort and vision
B Active protein can cause reduced lens comfort
C Denatured protein can cause red eye reactions

D Protein binds to soft lens surfaces as well as entering the matrix of the lens

E Protein-removing tablets are only effective on active proteins

Question 10.7
Which of the following solution properties has the least effect on initial comfort?

A Low pH

B Viscosity

C Tonicity

D Preservative concentration

E High pH

Question 10.8
According to the health belief model, which of the following statements is true?

A Compliance will be enhanced if an individual is less susceptible to developing the medical condition

B Compliance will be enhanced if the individual believes the medical condition is not serious

C A patient has more opportunities not to comply with a procedure, than to follow it

D Non-compliance is more likely when there are fewer reasons not to follow instructions

E A and C only

Question 10.9
Amongst student contact lens wearers, which of the following is the least commonly practised activity?

A Protein-removal cleaning

B Hand-washing

C Lens case cleaning

D Surfactant cleaning

E Lens disinfection

Question 10.10
Which of the following statements is false?

A Cleaning and rinsing together removes 99 per cent of micro-organisms

B Multi-purpose solutions can contain cleaning and protein removing properties

C Wetting solutions encourage an even distribution of tears over the lens on insertion

D Soft lens cases can be safely rinsed with tap water and allowed to air dry

E A non-wetting RGP lens can result from over-polishing during manufacture

References

1 Christie, C. L. and Meyler, J. G. (1997) Contemporary contact lens care products. *Contact Lens & Anterior Eye* **20S:** S11–S17.

2 Christie, C. L. (1999) Solutions: same or different? *Optician* **218: 5717** 20–24.

3 Long, B. (1998) Disinfection standards for contact lenses. *Optician* **216: 5676** 32–33.

4 BS EN ISO 14729: 2001 14729 Ophthalmic Optics – Contact Lens Care Products – Microbiological requirements and test methods for products and regimens for hygienic management of contact lenses.

5 Fletcher, E.L. and Brennan, N.A. (1993) The effect of solution tonicity on the eye. *Clin Exp Optom* **76:1** 17–21.

6 Harris, M.G., Higa, C.K., Lacey, L. L. and Barnhart, L.A. (1990) The pH of aerosol saline solution. *Optom Vis Sci* **67:2** 84–88.

7 Franklin, V., Tighe, B. and Tongue, S. (1995) Disclosure – the true story of multi-purpose solutions. *Optician* **209: 5500** 25–28.

8 Paugh, J. R., Brennan, N. A and Efron, N. (1988) Ocular response to hydrogen peroxide. *Am J Optom Physiol Opt* **65:2** 91–98.

9 Jones, L., Davies, I. and Jones, D. (1993) Effect of hydrogen peroxide neutralisation on the fitting characteristics of Group IV disposable contact lenses. *JBCLA* **16:4** 135–140

10 Seal, D.V, Kirkness, C.M. *et al.* (1999) *Acanthamoeba* keratitis in Scotland: Risk factors for contact lens wearers. *Contact Lens & Anterior Eye* **22:2** 58–68.

11 Claydon, B. E. and Efron, N. (1994) Non-compliance in general health care. *Ophthalmic Physiol Opt* **14:3** 257–264.

12 Claydon, B.E. and Efron, N. (1994) Non-compliance in contact lens wear. *Ophthalmic Physiol Opt* **14:4** 356–364.

13 Sokol, J.L. *et al.* (1990) A study of patient compliance in a contact lens-wearing population. *CLAO Journal* **16:3** 209–213.

14 Radford, C.F., Woodward, E.G. and Stapelton, F. (1993) Contact lens hygiene compliance in a university population. *JBCLA* **16:3** 105–111.

11
Extended wear

Introduction

Ever since contact lenses were first fitted, some patients have either chosen to sleep in them or been advised by doctors and optometrists to sleep in them.

Many of the first glass haptic lenses fitted, by, for example, the Mullers in the 1880s, were worn for up to one to two years at a time, and the literature contains many more reports of patients wearing both haptic and hard corneal lenses on an extended wear basis prior to 1974.[1] It was John de Carle, working in London, who first popularized hydrogel extended wear with the development of the Permalens. In 1981 hydrogel extended wear was approved by the Food and Drug Administration (FDA) in the US for cosmetic correction and the aggressive advertising and popularity of this modality led to its widespread acceptance in that country. Hydrogel extended wear lenses were typically worn for up to thirty days then removed, cleaned and reinserted. By 1985 an estimated four million patients were wearing extended wear lenses in the US.

In Europe demand has had a far less significant influence and the relative absence of extended wear advertising has led to fewer patients. Time will tell whether this will change with the availability of silicone hydrogel materials or whether such materials will be used primarily as 'problem-solving' lenses or for refitting existing hydrogel extended lens wearers.

The early extended wear research was carried out in an intuitive clinical manner with patient success being judged by the ability to continue to wear the lenses. As the 1980s progressed, the scientific interest in the mechanics and physiology of extended wear increased. In particular, there was an increased understanding of the oxygen needs of the cornea and the effect of oxygen depletion to that structure.

It is now well established that lack of oxygen to the eye leads to corneal swelling (oedema). During normal closed-eye sleep the cornea swells by an average of 4 per cent. It is capable, however, of recovering 8 per cent of swelling during the day and this became the target for hydrogel lenses. The landmark study by Holden and Mertz in 1984 defined the levels of oxygen needed to avoid corneal oedema[2] (Table 11.1). Further studies have shown the inability of the extended wear lenses fitted at that time to meet these needs. While hydrogel materials are unable to achieve the criteria of zero swelling with overnight wear, some come close to the 8 per cent level (0 residual swell) and gained regulatory approval for extended wear.

Modern rigid gas-permeable lenses (RGPs) and silicone hydrogels (Si-H) are, however, able to allow sufficient oxygen to the eye to achieve the zero swelling criteria. Nevertheless, it is important to remember the closed eye environment differs from the normal open eye in several key factors (Table 11.2).

As well as the issue of corneal hypoxia, early non-disposable hydrogel extended wear was also associated with inflammatory reactions due to long-term deposit build up, and toxic reactions due to the intensive cleaning procedures required after

- Available oxygen drops from 155 mmHg (atmospheric) to 55 mmHg (palpebral conjunctival capillaries)
- Corneal demand for oxygen increases
- Lens temperature increases about 2°C
- pH drops from 7.45 to 7.25
- Tear osmolarity decreases from 310-318 mOsm/kg to 285 mOsm/kg

Table 11.2
Closed eye environment.

thirty nights of wear. The introduction of weekly replaced disposable lenses in 1987 allowed these two issues to be resolved.

Further increases in the size of the extended wear market followed, particularly in the US. Disposable extended wear shows fewer overall complications, fewer unscheduled appointments and fewer patient symptoms than conventional extended wear lenses.[3] This was due primarily to the increased replacement frequency resulting in few allergy-based reactions. The incidence of corneal infection with disposable EW remained the same, although reports have suggested that the severity of the infection is less than that with non-disposable EW.[3]

The growth of the extended wear market in the US was curtailed in 1989 with the publication and popularization of a landmark study by Poggio and Schein.[4] This was sponsored by the Contact Lens Institution (CLI), an industry trade association. The study showed extended wear patients to have an incidence of keratitis of 20.9 per 10 000 patient years, compared to 4.1 per 10 000 for soft daily wear patients. The relative risk of developing microbial keratitis (MK) was shown to be increased by factors such as smoking and wearing lenses for more than six consecutive nights. The

	0% DW oedema	4% overnight oedema	0% EW residual oedema
Critical Dk/t_{avg} (x10^{-9}) @20°C	24.1	87.0	34.3
Critical EOP (% atmospheric O_2)	9.9	17.9	12.1

Table 11.1
Critical corneal oxygen requirements.[2]

Author	Year	Annualized incidence per 10 000				Relative risk of EW hydrogel to DW hydrogel
		DW RGP	DW hydrogel	EW RGP	EW hydrogel	
Poggio *et al*	1989	4.0	4.1	–	20.9	5.09
MacRae *et al*	1991	6.8	5.2	18.2	23.9	4.59
Benjamin	1991	1.1	2.1	4.2	8.8	4.2
Nilsson and Montan	1994	1.21	0.51	–	3.12	6.12
Schein *et al*	1989	–	–	–	–	12.6
Dart *et al*	1991	–	–	–	–	5.78
Cheng *et al*	1999	1.1	3.5	–	20	5.72

Table 11.3
Incidence and relative risk of microbial keratitis for different lens modalities.

relative risks of hydrogel extended wear versus daily wear have been verified in several studies since the original CLI study (Table 11.3), although Nilsson[5] showed a significant reduced incidence of the condition in Scandinavia.

Despite the low incidence rates (about 0.2 per cent) the Poggio and Schein study gained significant media coverage and reduced overall confidence in the modality. The study also led the FDA to recommend in 1989 that extended wear be limited to no more than seven days and six nights of continuous wear without removal of lenses for cleaning and disinfection. The FDA have recently approved silicone hydrogel lenses for up to 30 nights of extended wear.

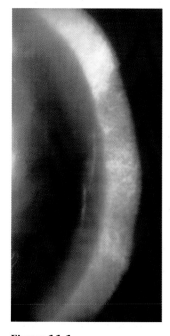

Figure 11.1
Striae resulting from hypoxia and corneal oedema (courtesy of CCLRU).

Current status

The relative risks of extended versus daily wear have been verified in many studies since the original Poggio and Schein study (Table 11.3). The incidence of complications, however, is less frequently studied and the Nilsson and Montan study[5] showed a significant reduced incidence of the condition in Scandinavia. Disposable extended wear has been shown to be beneficial over conventional extended wear, with careful patient selection and close follow-up.[3,6] This is due to the advantages of more frequent lens replacement and the avoidance of lens care solutions. However, hydrogel lenses have limited oxygen transmissibility, which can result in corneal hypoxia and the associatied clinical signs of striae (Figure 11.1), folds, microcysts and vascularization (Figure 11.2).

RGP extended wear has a number of advantages over the use of soft hydrogel lenses, notably, enhanced oxygen transmissibility and an active tear pump mechanism. These properties allow the issue of hypoxia to be addressed, with a resultant reduction in the risk of hypoxia related complications. Several disadvantages, however, have limited the more widespread use of this modality, with the main issue being comfort, lens binding resulting from changes in the tear film during sleep (Figure 11.3) and 3 and 9 o'clock staining.

Silicone hydrogel lenses were developed with the goal of addressing the limitations of oxygen transmission of hydrogel lenses and making extended wear a safer and more successful wearing modality.

Figure 11.4 shows typical silicone hydrogel chemistry where polydimethylsiloxanes (the silicone element) are attached to NVP (the hydrogel element)

through a cross-linking polymer. Unlike conventional hydrogels, silicone hydrogel oxygen permeability increases as the water content decreases. Increasing the silicone content may bring the benefit of increased oxygen permeability but will also decrease wettability and increase lipid interaction. Consequently, silicone hydrogel lenses have

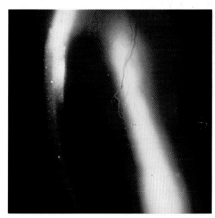

Figure 11.2
Microcysts and neovascularization in a long-term aphakic extended wear patient (courtesy of Lyndon Jones).

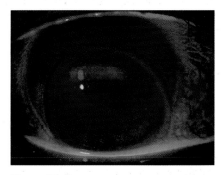

Figure 11.3
Lens binding following overnight wear with an RGP lens (photography by Lyndon Jones, copyright Bausch & Lomb).

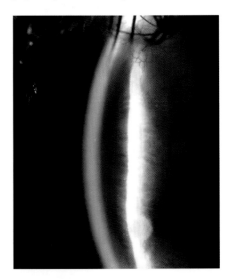

Figure 11.4
Representation of typical silicone hydrogel chemistry.

to be surface treated using gas plasma techniques. This has resulted in minimal protein deposition although there is still a tendency for lipid deposition.

Transmissibilities are such that incremental overnight corneal swelling with lens wear should be eliminated or significantly reduced. This was the primary design goal and studies confirm that overnight swelling is typically no greater than that measured with no lens wear. This is a significant breakthrough in material design with the result that the vast majority of wearers will show no signs of lens-induced hypoxia. Silicone hydrogel extended wear is not, however, complication free.[7,8]

Silicone hydrogel materials are approximately three times as stiff as hydrogel materials and will, therefore, give rise to more negative pressure under the lens during blinks than more flexible materials such as HEMA or etafilcon A. This may increase the incidence of mechanical arcuate lesions (Figure 11.5) with these materials as well as a more mechanically related papillary conjunctivitis (CLPC) which can result in discontinuations. 'Mucin balls' (Figure 11.6) are more frequently observed with silicone hydrogel lenses. Frequency increases the longer the period of extended wear and they are more likely to present in

eyes with steeper corneal curvature.[9] It is felt they are not detrimental to contact lens wear with no intervention required, assuming vision is not compromised.

Inflammatory responses can manifest as different adverse events. Contact lens acute red eye (CLARE), contact lens peripheral ulcer (CLPU) (Figure 11.7) and other infiltrative events can occur.[7,8] A specific guide has been designed to support the diagnosis and management of the full range of infiltrative conditions (Figure 11.8).

Whether silicone hydrogels result in a significant reduction in infectious keratitis when compared to hydrogel lenses has yet to be determined. If corneal oedema and the associated detrimental effect on epithelial integrity are the key risk factors, then it is reasonable to predict a reduction of infection rates. However, this reduction has not been noted with RGP EW lenses in one study (MacRae *et al*,[10] Table 11.3) which have comparable oxygen transmissibility to silicone hydrogel lenses.

Patient selection

Extended wear contact lenses are beneficial for many patients and there is no doubt that patients are interested in the convenience of

this lens wearing option especially if endorsed by their eye care professional. The benefits are particularly evident with many occupations such as doctors and nurses on night duty and those in the armed forces, in addition to certain hobbies, which make the management of daily wear lenses impractical. Infant or elderly aphakes are further examples of those who may also benefit from extended wear lenses, by overcoming handling and vision limitations.

However, this lens modality needs to be treated with respect in view of the greater incidence of overall complications as well as the risk of infectious keratitis. It is important, therefore, that a full explanation of the risks and benefits of extended wear are provided objectively, putting the patient in a position to make an informed choice. If the patient accepts this increased risk compared to daily wear, then the practitioner has to decide on the best course of action. There are three possibilities:
• Refuse to fit the patient regardless of physiological suitability. In this case the

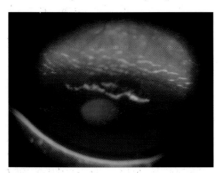

Figure 11.5
SEAL lesion resulting from contact lens wear (courtesy of Lyndon Jones).

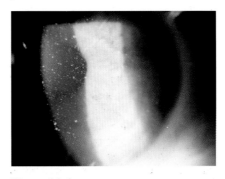

Figure 11.6
'Mucin balls' between lens and cornea in Si-H extended wear.

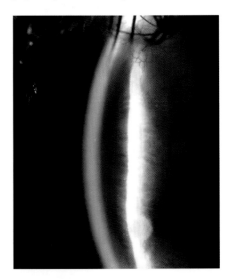

Figure 11.7
CLPU observed in extended wear patient (courtesy of David Ruston).

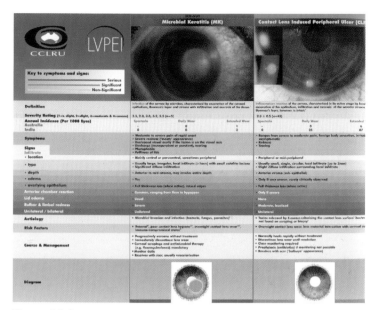

Figure 11.8
CCLRU/LVPEI guide to corneal infiltrative conditions.

patient might go to another practitioner who does not explain the risks and benefits and who might not take the care required to manage the modality.

• Refer the patient to a colleague who is more experienced in fitting and managing this modality or fit under supervision until more confident.

• Proceed with the evaluation of suitability and, if the patient is suitable, fit. This course of action maintains the relationship bet-

ween practitioner and patient and allows the practitioner to offer a total contact lens service.

Instrumentation

The instrumentation required for fitting contact lenses for extended wear is essentially the same as for basic contact lens fitting. However, it is vital that the slit-lamp biomicroscope has good optics and high magnification for viewing subtle corneal changes – in particular, striae, folds and microcysts. As with any form of contact lens practice, grading scales will allow more objective observation and recording of baseline tissue appearance prior to lens fitting.

It is important to monitor corneal distortion secondary to hypoxia in both RGP and soft contact lens wearers. The keratometer provides some, but rather limited, information in this regard. Keratoscopy can also play a useful role in monitoring corneal distortion. As for any contact lens, the presence of a normal, stable, tear film is important. The practitioner must, therefore, have access to instrumentation that permits tear assessment for both initial assessment and monitoring. In clinical practice, basic tear quality is best assessed by employing a non-invasive technique such as the use of the tearscope in conjunction with the slit-lamp.

Even with Hi-Dk RGP lenses and silicone hydrogel soft lenses, extended wear can

reduce oxygen levels to a level that results in corneal hypoxia and oedema in a small percentage of patients. Corneal oedema can be visualized through slit-lamp observation of striae, folds and, to some extent, microcysts. In routine clinical practice this is the best method for detecting corneal oedema. It can also be measured objectively as a function of the change in corneal thickness as this reflects the degree of swelling. The relative thickness of the cornea may be measured using a pachometer (Figure 11.9).

Since the overnight wear of a contact lens can result in greater significant adverse events, it is incumbent upon the practitioner to select candidates more carefully for extended wear. This involves careful pre-assessment but ultimately lens trial, which allows optimal fit, and frequent monitoring is required to establish physiological response.

Techniques

History and symptoms
The first stage in extended wear fitting, as in any contact lens fitting, is to get a full history and symptoms from the patient.

In extended wear fitting it is particularly important to fully understand and explore the reasons for the patient wanting overnight lens wear. Is it because the patient truly needs to sleep in lenses (e.g. occupational need) or has interest been generated by consumer advertising alone? Has the patient failed in other lens modalities and does he/she think that this may be a more appropriate form of contact lens wear? General laziness or failure to return for aftercare would be considered as contraindications to extended wear. High standards of patient hygiene are required, and consideration must also be made of the home or work environment

Ocular and general health must be questioned; for example, diabetes would be considered by many as a contraindication for extended wear but acceptable for daily wear.

Open questioning techniques should be used throughout the process to identify the patient needs. It is the obligation of the practitioner to ensure that the patient fully understands the risks and benefits of their chosen modality. The patient must also understand the importance of self-monitoring of their eyes and calling their

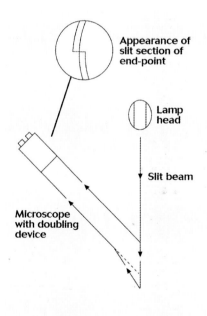

Figure 11.9
Optical principle of pachometry.

practitioner if there are any unusual findings or changes from the norm.

Although the absolute risk of developing a serious adverse reaction to extended wear lenses is small, the relative risk in comparison to daily wear is significant with hydrogel and RGP lenses and unknown at this time with silicone hydrogel lenses. The patient must understand this and the use of a written and signed acknowledgement form is to be recommended. As in all contact lens practice, the practitioner should fully record the outcome of the discussion with the patient.

Initial examination

Once the history and symptoms have been completed, the next stage is to carry out a detailed examination of the anterior segment to check for suitability of the patient for contact lens wear.

Overnight wear of contact lenses puts the cornea in a more stressful environment when compared to daily wear. It is, therefore, important to check that there are no contraindications at all to the wearer. It is possible that patients who may be borderline cases in terms of suitability, could be successful in daily wear lenses, but these patients should not be fitted with extended wear.

Particular aspects to be considered are: a stable tear film, no corneal staining, full blinking, minimal conjunctival hyperaemia, and minimal follicles or papillae on the tarsal plate. A recommended 'pre-health' checklist is shown in Table 11.4.

Keratometric assessment, covered in Chapter 3, should be taken to provide baseline data in the cornea of the soft extended wear patient, and fitting information for the RGP extended wear patient. The keratometer reflex should be regular and if keratoscopy is to be carried out, the cornea should show a regular contour with no distortion or warpage.

The practitioner's next responsibility is then to ensure that the patient is physiologically suitable for extended wear which can be achieved from lens trial.

Lens fitting

The basic principles of extended wear lens fitting are the same as for daily wear and have been covered in Chapters 5 and 6 for soft and hard lenses respectively. Maximizing oxygen supply to the eye in addition to adequate tear exchange to remove post-lens debris should be prime considerations.

Characteristic	Requirement
Comfort	Grade 3 (comfortable) or better
Subjective vision rating	Grade 3 (good) or better
Visual acuity	Within one line of best spectacle acuity
Hypoxic effects	No microcysts or vacuoles* No striae or signs of visible oedema
Limbal vascularization	<0.5mm vessel penetration
Corneal staining	None**
Endothelial polymegethism	≤Grade 1
Changes in corneal curvature	No irregular corneal distortion or warpage**
Infiltrates	None**
Bulbar and palpebral conjunctival redness	≤Grade 1
Palpebral conjunctival papillae	≤Grade 1
Conjunctival staining	≤Grade 1

*Existing wearers may show some degree of microcysts, vacuoles or corneal distortion or warpage and clinical judgement should be used to assess suitability for fitting
**Extended wear lenses should not be fitted until staining or infiltrates are resolved

Table 11.4
Pre-fit checklist on ocular health as recommended by Brennan and Coles.[11]

In hydrogel lens fitting, the fit should err on the looser side of normal as observed on push-up test while maintaining corneal coverage and good comfort. This enhances the removal of metabolic debris from under the lens surface. Silicone hydrogel fitting is more critical due to the relative stiffness of current materials with poor lens fit/discomfort being the primary reason for discontinuations in one study.[12] Careful observation of edge alignment of the lens to the bulbar conjunctiva should be made during biomicroscopic examination, as 'edge-fluting' can be a significant reason for poor comfort and an unsuccessful fit. Primary gaze post-blink movement should be 0.2–0.3mm. Excessive movement will result in discomfort.

RGP lenses should be fitted to achieve an optimum fit to avoid 3 and 9 o'clock staining and lens binding. Fitting as close as possible to alignment to achieve equal lens bearing across the cornea reduces the risk of lens binding. In particular, if the lens is too tight in the mid periphery this will increase the risk of lens binding. Lack of tear exchange will cause an increase in tear viscosity. Other design considerations differentiating RGP extended wear from daily wear include increasing lens diameter to help stabilize the fit and increasing peripheral clearance to help in avoiding lens binding.

It is critical with extended wear fitting that lenses be thoroughly cleaned and disinfected on removal, if they are to be reinserted. In extended wear, weekly replaced single-use disposables and silicone hydrogel lenses overcome this need. However, the latter necessitates the need for a longer period of continuous wear (up to one month) if lens care solutions are to be avoided.

Lens adaptation

In the authors' opinion, it is important that patients adapt fully to their lenses on a daily wear basis before starting to sleep in them.

Typically, at least one week of daily wear should be completed for soft lenses with the wearing time being gradually increased each day in the normal manner. Of course the build up will be more gradual for the novice RGP wearer.

If the patient is being fitted with silicone hydrogel lenses or disposable hydrogel extended wear lenses, it is particularly important that he/she understands the importance of cleaning and disinfecting the lenses during this adaptation period and that they be given full instruction in lens maintenance, even though they will not be required to do this once they are wearing the lenses on single use extended wear basis (i.e. disposal on removal).

Once the patient has built up to all day wear they should, ideally, attend an aftercare appointment before commencing overnight wear. At this aftercare appointment, the practitioner should evaluate the extent to which the patient has adapted to lens wear.

Practitioners should be cautious about overnight wear if there are any visible signs of lack of adaptation to the lenses during daily wear. In particular, signs of oedema, conjunctival hyperaemia, palpebral changes, corneal infiltrates or corneal staining, whether resulting from desiccation or mechanical insult, as well as lens binding.

If the eye is clear and the patient appears to have fully adapted to daily lens wear then they may proceed with the first night of overnight wear. The practitioner should instruct their patient to remove the lens if there is any pain or significant redness of the eye, either during the night or upon waking. They should be told to check for lens movement on eye opening and ocular lubricants can be recommended for morning use to encourage movement and flushing of debris from beneath the lens. It is also important to schedule a follow-up appointment for the morning after the first night of extended wear.

It must be emphasized, however, that the ability of any patient to wear extended wear, soft contact lenses for one week to one month does not assure continued success indefinitely. Regular and ongoing aftercare visits are essential for patients wearing extended wear lenses.

First aftercare appointment

The appointment after the first night of extended wear should be made as early as possible in the morning. This is when the cornea will have its most stressed appearance and is, therefore, the optimal time for slit-lamp examination regardless of the lens type worn. On lens removal it is critically important to look immediately for signs of corneal oedema, in particular, striae and endothelial folds. This is to ensure that these

signs are not missed. For example, striae will typically be observed only within four hours of awakening. Table 11.5 summarizes the relationship between the level of oedema and slit-lamp observation.

The examination routine should follow the normal aftercare pattern (see Chapter 9) with particular attention paid in the history and symptoms section to the comfort and vision of the lens upon eye opening and then the speed of resolution of any symptoms, which ought to be quite rapid.

The assessment of lens fit should show free-moving lenses with no sign of lens binding. Visual acuity in the lenses should not show any difference from that obtained before the first night of extended wear.

All extended wear patients should be instructed to respond to any signs or symptoms quickly and appropriately. Patients should be advised to remove the lenses immediately if they experience any pain, red eye or blurred vision, and call their practitioner for advice. This availability of immediate advice should be supported further by supplying patients with an after-hours emergency contact. Remember, early symptoms of potentially serious problems can be subtle; foreign body sensation is frequently the earliest symptom of microbial keratitis.

Educating the patient as to appropriate self-management can enhance the success and safety of contact lens wear.

It is important that all practice staff who may receive calls from contact lens patients understand the appropriate action. On lens removal if the patient's signs or symptoms persist, an urgent appointment with the practitioner should be made. It has to be remembered that serious adverse responses can develop within 24 hours.

Patients should be instructed to bring their lenses, their case and any solutions used to the appointment. As with daily wear contact lens users, all extended lens wearers should be advised to have an up-to-date pair of spectacles for use as necessary.

On awakening each morning the extended lens wearer should carry out a self-

Key points

- The risks and benefits of extended wear should be discussed between the patient and practitioner to help enable an informed choice to be made.
- Careful patient selection and lens trial is of vital importance. Extended wear lenses should only be considered for ideal contact lens patients.
- It is critical that extended wear patients are both carefully and frequently monitored throughout their contact lens wearing life, with regular aftercare checks.
- All extended wear patients should be instructed to self-monitor their eyes daily, and to understand the procedures to follow should any variations from the norm be observed.

assessment:
- Do my eyes look good?
- Do my eyes feel good?
- Do my eyes see good?

If any of these questions are answered in the negative, then lenses should immediately be removed and the decision tree followed as outlined in Chapter 9.

Ongoing aftercare

Following a successful fitting and first overnight wear the patient should be monitored after one week, and thereafter every three months or more frequently as required. All appointments should be made as early as possible in the morning.

As with all contact lens wearers, a full eye examination and ophthalmoscopy should be undertaken at least every two years or sooner if symptoms suggest a non-contact lens-related problem.

Interpretation of findings

Results from patient discussion, measurement and observation all need to be taken into account in deciding the course of action to be taken. Table 11.6 summarizes the main complications seen in extended wear patients and recommends management options. Many conditions are less frequently observed during daily wear follow-up and all forms of continuing education on extended wear are to be encouraged to ensure appropriate

Oedema	1–4%	5–7%	8–10%	>10%
Striae (no)	0	1–3	5–8	≥9
Folds (no)	0	0	1–3	≥4

Table 11.5
Critical assessment of corneal oedema.

Observation	Possible cause	Action required
1–3 striae • within 4 hours of awakening	Mild stromal oedema due to closed eye	Monitor for persistence later in the day Increase oxygen supply
• present >4 hours after awakening	Excessive oedema	Change to daily wear
≥4 striae and/or folds	Excessive oedema	Increase oxygen supply Change to daily wear
10–30 microcysts	Mild corneal hypoxia and/or hypercapnia	Increase oxygen supply* Monitor more frequently
>30 microcysts	Excessive corneal hypoxia and/or hypercapnia	Increase oxygen supply* Change to daily wear
Vascularization (note: most commonly seen in superior cornea initially)	Long-term hypoxia with hydrogel contact lens wear	Increase oxygen supply Change to daily wear Refit with RGP or silicone hydrogel
CLPC (contact lens-associated papillary conjunctivitis)	Deposit build-up on lenses (especially denatured protein)	Replace lenses and consider frequent replacement thereafter
Corneal staining • desiccation	Pervaporization of tears	Increase replacement frequency Try alternative material Use ocular lubricants
• 3 and 9 o'clock	Compromised RGP fit Incomplete blinking Poor surface wetting	Modify fit Blinking exercises New RGP lenses
• arcuate lesions (e.g. SEAL)	Hypoxia under upper lid Mechanical Poor lens fit	Increase oxygen supply Use material with lower elasticity Improve fit. Change lens design
CLARE (contact lens acute red eye)	Poor tear exchange Tight lens fit Bound lens Exotoxins from bacteria	Loosen fit. Try alternative lens design Loosen fit Improve fit, try ocular lubricants, change lens design Improve lens hygiene, increase lens replacement frequency
Corneal infiltrate (non-staining)	Hypoxia Poor tear exchange Tight lens fit Solution reaction	Remove lens and allow to resolve Increase oxygen supply Loosen fit. Try alternative lens design Loosen fit Change solution regimen
CLPU (contact lens peripheral ulcer)	Exotoxins from bacteria	Remove lens and monitor over 24 hours If symptoms and signs increase: immediate referral
Infectious ulcer	Microbial invasion of cornea	Immediate referral

* Note: when refitting with higher Dk/t lens, the number of microcysts may increase prior to being reduced or eliminated

Table 11.6
Management guidelines of extended wear complications.

recognition and management when prescribing this modality.

Summary

It is important to view the issues of extended wear in perspective. Although there may be an increased risk of microbial keratitis compared to daily wear, there is significantly less risk of loss of best corrected visual acuity when compared to other surgical forms of vision correction, e.g. Lasik.[13,14]

Extended wear is not a suitable modality for everybody but recent material developments may increase success rates. It can be the best choice for others – especially those with specific vocational or recreational demands and medical indications. Increased marketing of this lens wearing option will no doubt lead to increased interest by patients. If the need for extended wear is established it is better for the practitioner to manage responsibly rather than merely to say no. Informed choice and continuous careful monitoring are of the utmost importance.

New lens materials, in the form of silicone hydrogels, have resulted in a significant improvement in satisfying the physiological requirements of the cornea during eye closure in that hypoxic-related complications should no longer be a feature of extended wear for the majority of patients. However, current designs are not without limitations and complications which require appropriate recognition and management. This may involve the use of hydrogel disposables, RGP lenses, moving to daily wear or, in the future, the use of therapeutic agents by contact lens practitioners. Additional fitting parameters would also be beneficial to allow more optimal fitting.

Although the aetiology of microbial keratitis is complex, a significant risk factor is contact lens-induced hypoxia as well as mechanical and inflammatory events. Although initial results are promising, whether hypoxia elimination alone is enough to reduce the incidence of MK can only be determined by population based studies or post-marketing surveillance following widespread use of these products in the market. Regardless, the importance of patient selection, optimal lens fitting and comprehensive/regular follow-up remains the same.

Question 11.1
Which of the following statements regarding the closed eye environment is false?
A Tear pH becomes more acidic
B Tear osmolarity decreases
C Available oxygen decreases
D Corneal demands for oxygen decreases
E Lens temperature increases

Question 11.2
The critical average transmissibility to allow 4 per cent or less overnight oedema is?
A 34.3
B 87.0
C 24.1
D 120.0
E 67.4

Question 11.3
During normal closed eye sleep (i.e. without contact lens wear) the cornea swells by an average of:
A 0 per cent
B 2 per cent
C 4 per cent
D 8 per cent
E 20 per cent

Question 11.4
Which of the following signs in a daily contact lens wearer would not contraindicate switching to extended wear?
A Corneal staining
B >grade 1 bulbar conjunctival hyperaemia
C Corneal oedema
D >grade 1 palpebral papillae redness
E Small, non-staining corneal scar

Question 11.5
Which of the following instruments cannot be used to observe and/or measure significant amounts of corneal oedema?
A Optical pachometer
B Slit-lamp biomicroscope
C Tearscope
D Ultrasonic pachometer
E Keratometer

Question 11.6
Which fitting and aftercare schedule is recommended for extended wear patients?
A 1 week DW/1 night EW/1 week review/3 month routine
B 1 week EW/4 week review/3 month routine
C 1 night EW/1 week review/6 month routine
D 1week DW/1 night EW/1 week review/6 month routine
E 1 week DW/1 week EW/3 month routine

Question 11.7
Which of the following observations would be made in the presence of 6 per cent corneal oedema due to soft lens wear?
A Central corneal clouding
B Two folds
C Two striae
D Significantly reduced visual acuity
E Five striae

Question 11.8
Which of the following conditions is less likely to be observed with silicone hydrogel materials when compared to hydrogel lenses?
A SEAL lesions
B 'Mucin balls'
C Corneal oedema
D Infiltrates
E CLARE

Question 11.9
Appropriate management approach for CLPU is:
A Loosen fit
B Increase oxygen supply
C Change solution regime
D Cease lens wear, monitor and refer if signs/symptoms increase
E Refer immediately

Question 11.10
Appropriate management for suspected infectious ulcer is?
A Remove lens and allow to resolve
B Refer immediately
C Refit and increase oxygen supply
D Use ocular lubricants
E Change solution regimen

References

1 Young, G. (1985) Overview on rigid lens extended wear before 1984. *JBCLA* **8:2** 71–77.
2 Holden, B.A. and Mertz, G.W. (1984) Critical oxygen levels to avoid corneal oedema for daily and extended wear. *Invest Ophthal Vis Sci* **25:** 1161–1167.
3 Poggio, E.G. and Abelson, M. (1993) Complications and symptoms in disposable extended wear lenses compared with conventional soft daily wear and soft extended wear lenses. *CLAO Journal* **19:1** 31–39.
4 Poggio, E.G. and Schien, O.D. (1989) The incidence of ulcerative keratitis among wearers of daily wear and extended wear soft contact lenses. *N Eng J Med* **321:** 779–783.
5 Nilsson, E.G. and Montan, P.G. (1994) The hospitalized cases of contact lens induced keratitis in Sweden and their relation to lens type and wear schedule: results of a three year retrospective study. *CLAO Journal* **20:2** 97–101.
6 Hamano, H. (1994) A study of the complications induced by conventional and disposable contact lenses. *CLAO Journal* **20:2** 103–7.
7 Edwards, K. (1999) Complications of hydrogel extended wear. *Optician* **218:5717** 26–30.
8 Holden, B. (2000) Adverse events and

infections: which ones and how many? In: Sweeney, D. F. (ed). *Silicone Hydrogels, the rebirth of continuous wear contact lenses.* Butterworth-Heinemann, 150–213

9 Dumbleton, K. (2000) Clinical characterisation of spherical post-lens debris associated with lotrafilcon high-Dk silicone lenses. *CLAO Journal* **26:4** 186–192.

10 MacRae, S. (1991) Corneal ulcer and adverse reaction rates in pre-market contact lens studies. *Am J Ophthalmol* **111:** 457–465.

11 Brennan, N. and Coles, C. (2000) Where do silicone hydrogels fit into everyday practice? In: Sweeney, D.F. (ed). *Silicone Hydrogels, the rebirth of continuous wear contact lenses.* Butterworth-Heinemann, 235–70.

12 Long, *et al.*(2000) Six months of in-practice experience with a high Dk Lotrafilcon A soft contact lens. *Contact Lens & Anterior Eye* **23:4** 112–118.

13 Cheng, K.H. (1999) Incidence of contact lens associated microbial keratitis and its related morbidity. *Lancet* **354:7** 179–183.

14 Waring, G.O. (1999) Lasik for myopia and astigmatism for 2,100 consecutive eyes using a Nidek EC-5000 Eximer laser. *Invest Ophthalmol Vis Sci* **40**: S588.

Further reading

Terry, R.L (1993) The CCLRU standards for success of daily and extended wear contact lenses. *Optician* **206:5430** 18–24.

Ruben, M. and Guillon, M. (1994) *Contact Lens Practice.* Chapman & Hall.

Sweeney, D.F. (2000) *Silicone Hydrogels, the rebirth of continuous wear contact lenses.* Butterworth-Heinemann.

12
Therapeutic contact lenses

Introduction

In general contact lens practice, there is no doubt that the most common indication for contact lens use is optical, i.e. the correction of ametropia.

However, this book would not be complete without paying attention to the use of contact lenses for therapeutic indications.

Hospital-based contact lens practitioners will have greater involvement in the use of contact lenses for therapeutic purposes. However, practitioners in general practice may be called upon to assist in the management of therapeutic contact lens wearers. In addition, they may be called upon to manage a patient attending for aftercare wearing a therapeutic lens.

It must be remembered that the very first contact lenses ever fitted in the 1880s were for therapeutic purposes. To this day, although scleral lenses still offer relief for a variety of pathological ocular conditions, soft lenses have gained more widespread use as bandage lenses. Initial success was limited due to low water content materials and thicker lens designs, hence a poor oxygen performance.

Today, practitioners have at their disposal more sophisticated soft lens materials, improved lens designs, and lens care options.

Silicone rubber lenses, collagen shields and rigid-gas permeable scleral lenses also have their applications. These developments, together with a better understanding of corneal physiology, have led to greater success with therapeutic lenses in a wide range of anterior segment pathologies.

With therapeutic contact lenses, principal aims include pain relief, mechanical protection and facilitation of wound healing. A more extensive list of functions is provided in Table 12.1

It is rare that therapeutic lenses are fitted on the basis of a single indicating factor; multiple aims are more commonplace in the presence of anterior segment pathology. For example, pain relief, mechanical protection and wound healing are frequently required in combination (Figure 12.1).

Although optimizing visual acuity may still be a desired objective, in diseased eyes it is often a secondary consideration.

The authors believe co-management of patients between ophthalmologists and contact lens practitioners is of great benefit to the patient receiving optimum care from the appropriate specialist. It is usual for both these services to be provided at the same hospital, requiring one visit by the patient.

However, shared-care opportunities are appropriate in some circumstances with experienced practitioners in general practice providing the contact lens service. Routine attendance at a hospital may not always be practical and the convenience of a local practice may be of great benefit to the patient. If a practitioner in private practice is to become involved in the management of therapeutic lens wearers, close liaison with the ophthalmologist is essential, with agreed guidelines on problem management.

Potential candidates for therapeutic lens wear are unique in contact lens fitting, as they possess numerous contraindications for contact lens wear. These can be either ocular in nature, for example dry eye, disrupted epithelium – or general in nature, for example, arthritic or diabetic patients.

Compared to cosmetic lens fitting to a healthy eye, the risk of fitting a lens to the already compromised eye is, of course, greater. Inducing a state of relative hypoxia

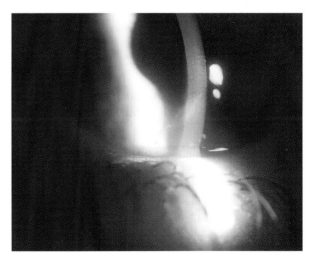

Figure 12.1
Paper cut to cornea. In this case a bandage lens would offer pain relief, promote epithelial healing and protection against the action of the lids (courtesy of Lyndon Jones).

Pain relief

Mechanical protection (cornea and lids)

To promote epithelial healing

Maintenance of hydration

Structural support

To seal corneal perforations

To improve visual acuity (distorted cornea)

Delivery of medication

Table 12.1
Functions of therapeutic contact lenses.

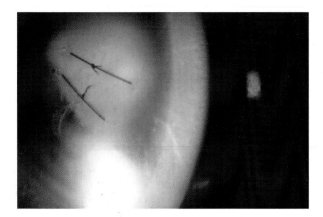

Figure 12.2
Following a penetrating injury a bandage lens could be used to protect the lid from proud suture ends (courtesy of A. J. Bron).

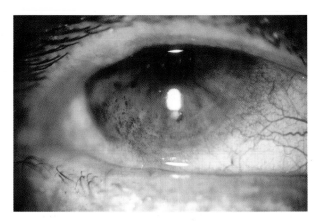

Figure 12.3
Rose bengal staining confirming a severe dry eye (courtesy of Lyndon Jones).

and possible mechanical trauma due to the presence of a lens can be problematic. Furthermore, altered tear film dynamics due to trapped debris, reduced nutrient circulation and reduced movement of bacteriostatic element can potentially further compromise the eye.

The balance between benefits and potential risks must be carefully considered before fitting a therapeutic lens. Careful patient monitoring and instruction on what to do if a problem arises are of utmost importance.

A range of contact lens types can be used for therapeutic purposes, including:
• Hydrogels
• Silicone hydrogels
• Silicone rubber lenses
• Collagen shields
• RGP corneal lenses
• Scleral lenses
• Scleral rings

The choice of lens type will depend upon the condition to be treated.

Silicone rubber lenses have been advocated in cases of lid abnormalities or dry eye, but there are inherent problems with adherence and deposition of the lens surface. In some cases a thicker lower water content hydrogel lens may perform the therapeutic role well. In addition, there may be a role for the use of a silicone hydrogel in these examples. In cases where the primary reason for the fitting is to improve visual acuity, for example corneal irregularity, a hard or rigid gas-permeable lens will most commonly be the best choice. The rigid lens forms a smooth refracting surface, with the liquid tear lens neutralizing any irregularities from the corneal surface.

The most common therapeutic indication for rigid lens fitting is keratoconus. Other conditions resulting in an irregular cornea such as epithelial dystrophy and post-surgical distortion may also benefit from RGPs. The goal of correcting the distorted cornea is to balance the fit of the lens with the amount of physical compromise that achieving that fit produces. From a management perspective, the goal is to achieve adequate vision without further damage to the already compromised cornea.

This type of lens fitting is beyond the scope of this chapter, which will concentrate on the more common use of hydrogel lenses for therapeutic purposes.

Even if a practitioner does not fit lenses for therapeutic purposes, all should have a working knowledge of the range of conditions appropriate for treatment with therapeutic lenses and what to do if an existing wearer presents at the practice.

Instrumentation

The basic instrumentation required for therapeutic lens fitting is the same as that needed to fit regular soft lenses (see Chapter 5). A number of additional features should, however, be considered when using these instruments.

Slit-lamp
The presence of an anterior segment disorder commonly renders the patient photophobic, so the ability to diffuse light and/or reduce the intensity of the slit-lamp beam is of particular value in minimizing patient discomfort.

In addition to using fluorescein stain, rose bengal can be used in assessment of the dry-eyed patient. When using 1 per cent rose bengal Minims, care should be taken to instil only the tiniest amount possible as it can cause great discomfort to the patient. Furthermore, the dye will also stain the lids and skin surrounding the eyes and is relatively persistent. Rose bengal staining is viewed under white or green light, staining dead tissue red (Figure 12.3).

Keratometer
As the keratometer only provides an estimation of corneal curvature based upon an approximate 3.2 mm cord of its surface, this is often of limited value when assessing a cornea in the presence of pathology.

Keratometry is often difficult in cases of corneal disease, and is generally not necessary for adequate fitting of soft bandage lenses. However, it may have a value in monitoring the progression of some conditions, for example, keratoconus and progressive corneal dystrophies.

Very steep or very flat K-readings can be a feature of distorted or scarred corneas. If desired, an adaptation to the standard keratometer can be made to permit the measurement of a wider range of K-readings than commonly experienced in routine practice.

In the presence of gross corneal distortion and the absence of any corneal graft, measuring K-readings of the fellow non-diseased eye can provide a useful guide.

The technique of keratoscopy allows a more comprehensive assessment of the corneal contour. Practitioners attempting to fit irregular corneas with contact lenses

Pathology	Site of disorder	Lens function	Lens choice	Approximate length of therapy	Comments
Recurrent erosion	Corneal epithelium	Pain relief Promotion of stable epithelium	High or mid-water content soft lens	2–3 months (often reoccurs)	Controversial use. Symptomatic patients only after treatment of MGD* and lubricate
Filamentary keratitis	Corneal epithelium	Pain relief	High or mid-water content soft lens	2 weeks	
Thygeson's superficial punctate keratitis	Corneal epithelium	Pain relief	High or mid-water content soft lens	1 month daily wear (may reoccur)	Use unpreserved solutions
Corneal perforation (Descemetocele)	Corneal epithelium	Splint/seal leak	High water content soft lens	<1 month in close liaison with ophthalmologist	Large diameter lens often required. Tighter fit
Bullous keratopathy	Corneal epithelium	Pain relief from lid interaction with ruptured bullae	Mid-water content soft lens or silicone hydrogel. Regular lens replacement	>12 months	Watch for vascularization. Cornea gradually scars over. Try to wean off lens as bullae subside
Chemical burns: Acid Alkali	Cornea Conjunctiva	Pain relief Promotion of stable epithelialization Maintenance of fornices	High water content soft lens with scleral ring Scleral lens	Variable (weeks/months) until epithelialization occurs	Copious irrigation prior to lens insertion
Stevens-Johnson syndrome	Conjunctiva	Pain relief Mechanical protection	Thick, medium water content soft lens	Indefinite	Selected cases only
Exposure keratitis	Lids	Maintenance of hydration Mechanical protection	Scleral lens DW Mid-water soft lens Silicone lens	Indefinite	Often tape lids at night
Entropion Trichiasis	Lids	Protection	Thin, mid-water content soft lens Regular replacement	Pending surgery	Watch lid hygiene
Severe dry eye	Tear film	Maintenance of hydration	Sealed RGP scleral lens Silicone lens	2–12 months ongoing	Strict hygiene and follow-up

*Meibomian gland dysfunction

Table 12.2
Indications for therapeutic lens wear.

may find a photokeratoscope of great value (see Chapter 3).

Techniques

As with all contact lens fittings, an initial examination is required to evaluate patient characteristics and document baseline pathology.

The success of therapeutic lens wear is influenced by the selection of appropriate pathological cases. Table 12.2 lists pathologies for which therapeutic contact lenses may

be indicated and suggests the lens of choice.

The pre-fitting assessment should include a detailed slit-lamp examination, grading and documenting all abnormalities of the anterior segment, including the anterior chamber. Particular attention should also be paid to the lid margins and tear film. In general terms these have been discussed in Chapter 1. In most cases, a bandage lens is worn on an extended-wear basis for a relatively short period of time (weeks/months), but the patient must have the capacity to detect a problem and to seek urgent assistance.

It is not uncommon in therapeutic lens fitting that the patient is unable to handle their lenses. This may be due to a problem of physical dexterity or an inability to see clearly enough.

In these cases, the practitioner must ensure that arrangements are made for the patient to be able to have lenses removed in cases of emergency. This can either be achieved through tuition of a spouse, neighbour, carer or health visitor.

When daily wear of therapeutic lenses is indicated, the patient's age, physical dexterity (for example, the patient may suffer from

High oxygen transmissibility

Parameter range:

  choice of BOZR

  choice of TD

Parameter stability

Deposit management

Economical

Table 12.3
Requirements of a therapeutic lens.

arthritis), comprehension and motivation must also be considered, although, as previously mentioned, 'patient suitability' has to be viewed more leniently once the need for a therapeutic lens is established.

The risks and benefits need to be weighed up by the prescribing practitioner.

Lens selection

The choice of lens will depend primarily upon the specific disorder for which the lens is being prescribed. The general requirements are considered below and summarized in Table 12.3.

Oxygen transmissibility

The primary requirement of any contact lens is that it provides minimal interference with corneal metabolism. This is of particular importance in therapeutic cases as it may be necessary for the lens to be worn for prolonged periods, including overnight wear, or an eye which is invariably already compromised. Furthermore, the need for a therapeutic lens is often immediate and there is no possibility for gradual adaptation to lens wear.

Hence, for hydrogel lens use, high water content lenses or thin, mid-water contact lenses are often lenses of first choice, to maximize oxygen transmissibility. The selection of lens water content and/or thickness will be dependent upon the corneal disorder being treated. For example, a thicker lens may be more desirable when the function is to act as a splint (as in descemetocele) or to cover an irregular corneal surface. The use of silicone hydrogels to maximize oxygen transmissibility further may also be indicated in therapeutic lens fitting.

Thicker lenses may also be desirable in some cases of tear-film instability to support

a more stable tear structure. A thinner lens is more appropriate in cases of epithelial disruption (for example, recurrent erosion).

Parameter range

The majority of 'bandage lenses' used are plano or near plano prescription. In most circumstances, soft lenses of standard total diameters 14.0 mm to 15.0 mm will suffice. Larger diameter lenses (15.5 mm to 20 mm) may be required where the specific function is to protect the limbus or prevent wound leakage at suture or incision sites.

Larger diameter lenses require flatter back optic zone radii to achieve the desired fit. The key point, as in all contact lens fitting, is to ensure that an adequate physical fit is obtained, albeit the practitioner may need to settle for an 'acceptable fit' rather than an 'ideal fit'.

Parameter stability

Another consideration in fitting therapeutic lenses is the stability of the lenses once in the eye. All hydrogel lenses dehydrate *in vivo* to some extent, and while this is not of concern to a patient with a normal tear film, a dry-eyed patient may be unable to wear some lens materials or designs. The practitioner should therefore have a range of different materials and designs to choose from.

Deposit management

Given the pathological condition of the eyes fitted with therapeutic lenses, it is clearly desirable to minimize deposit build-up on the lens surface. The ideal therapeutic lens would be deposit resistant. A more practical approach is to use disposable or frequent replacement lenses as long as an adequate fit can be obtained. Today, therapeutic

lenses are rarely cleaned and reinserted on the same patient.

Economical

The final requirement of a therapeutic lens, especially in these days of reducing healthcare spending, is that it be economical for the practitioner/hospital to use. Lens replacement can be required as frequently as hourly, daily or weekly. For example, a daily disposable lens is ideal in cases of vernal keratoconjunctivitis where the excess mucus coats the lens within hours. Frequent change of lens prevents the abnormal mucus forming plaques on the damaged corneal epithelial surface.

Lens fitting

Ideally, a well-fitting bandage lens should provide full corneal coverage and be centred, with adequate movement (0.3 mm to 0.5 mm with each blink) to allow clearance of debris. It is important for the lens fit to be stable, avoiding excessive movement, as this can cause discomfort or epithelial disruption. Stability can be enhanced by increasing the lens total diameter. A relatively steeper fit may be preferred in cases such as irregular topography, or where vaulting or splinting is desired (Figure 12.4). A steeper fit is also desirable for delivery of medication – the lens acting as a reservoir for medications.

Aftercare

The fit of a soft bandage lens to be worn on an extended wear basis should be assessed in the same manner as for soft lenses

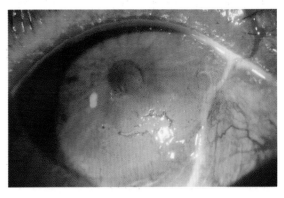

Figure 12.4
A bandage lens can act as a temporary splint with a leaking wound (courtesy of A. J. Bron).

generally as described in Chapter 5. Practitioners should be aware that the lens fit may change as the therapy progresses.

Visual acuity should be measured and recorded at each visit.

Routine instruction on how to insert and remove therapeutic lenses is rarely practical or indicated.

For all therapeutic lens wearers, it is vitally important that the practitioner ensures the patient is well instructed on both the need for good hygiene and what action to take if a problem arises. It may also be of benefit to explain to a relative or carer the important signs and symptoms that should be observed. Continued education at each aftercare visit reinforces the importance of the need for urgent action, especially with elderly patients, as they will almost inevitably find the effort and inconvenience of keeping an appointment even greater.

It is usual for a bandage lens to be worn on an extended wear basis, hence the lens fit and ocular status should be reviewed again after the first night of wear. However, in contrast to cosmetic extended wear, a bandage lens may not necessarily be removed at this appointment. Corneal health and progress of healing has to be monitored with the lens *in situ*, as the process of removal may disrupt the healing process (Figure 12.5). History and symptoms, visual acuity and a full slit-lamp examination with the lens *in situ* should be carried out.

The length of wear of the therapeutic lens and the frequency of aftercare will be dependent upon the underlying pathology (Table 12.2). Ongoing liaison with the ophthalmologist is of utmost importance.

Frequent appointments are usually indicated in the presence of active corneal pathology.

The length of time a therapeutic lens is required can vary greatly from as little as one hour to many months. Lenses should be replaced for reasons of loss, damage or deposition. It is common practice for lenses to be kept *in situ* until the desired aim has been achieved, and then discarded.

This is particularly apt in cases when epithelial wound healing is the aim. A minimum of six to eight weeks is required for hemidesmosomes to form once the superficial cells are in place. In contrast, in cases such as bullous keratopathy where the lens provides pain relief, regular lens removal and replacement is desired. In such cases the use of disposable lenses is beneficial. The silicone hydrogel lens has proved very successful in the management of this patient group.

In cases such as trichiasis, a lens is worn to protect the cornea until the appropriate surgery can be performed (Figure 12.6).

With therapeutic lenses, lens removal should be carried out with care. The lens can be floated off with saline irrigation to minimize trauma to the delicate epithelium.

Management of complications

Establishing success or failure criteria with a therapeutic lens is very difficult. For many, success can be measured in terms of subjective relief of pain. From a physiological standpoint, success can be judged by the corneal response to therapeutic lens coverage. The goal will vary according to the type and extent of pathology present.

Many of the potential complications of

therapeutic contact lens wear are identical to those that can occur with the use of extended wear lenses worn for cosmetic purposes.

However, the very fact that contact lenses are worn on an extended-wear basis on an already compromised eye places therapeutic lens wearers at particular risk of developing more serious complications. The risk can be further enhanced by additional factors such as diabetes, or the concurrent use of topical corticosteroids.

The patient should be informed of the benefits and risks of therapeutic lens wear, and be educated in the presentation of complications.

The practitioner should be aware that the incidence of infection among therapeutic lens wearers is greater than in cosmetic extended lens wearers and be especially vigilant. In view of the increased risk of microbial keratitis, ophthalmologists often prescribe antibiotics for prophylactic purposes, especially in the presence of an epithelial defect. Opinion is divided as to the prophylactic effect of topical antibiotic therapy, and practitioners should be aware of potential toxicity effects. As with any topical medication used concurrently with soft lenses the toxic effects can be minimized by using non-preserved drops in Minim form. If the medication is not available in non-preserved form, the use of disposable lenses, discarded weekly or less, can be an acceptable compromise.

Patients often benefit from the use of non-preserved wetting drops to insert upon waking and thereafter as required. The use of medication in ointment form is not appropriate because of the effect on lens wettability and vision.

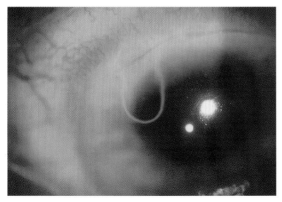

Figure 12.5
Slow-healing epithelium following chemical injury (acid) to the eye (courtesy of A. J. Bron).

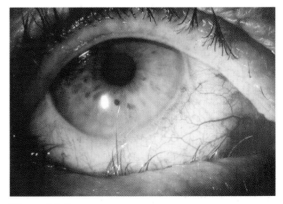

Figure 12.6
With trichiasis, a bandage lens is required to protect the cornea from the lashes (courtesy of A. J. Bron).

Patient related	Lens related
Severity of ocular pathology	Hypoxia
Concurrent dry eye	low water content
Concurrent topical corticosteroids	thick lens
Poor compliance	
ocular hygiene	Deposition
general hygiene	Mechanical insult
Poor general health	Poor fit
Lack of motivation	
Absence of carer	

Table 12.4
Factors associated with complications in therapeutic lens wear.

Lens-related effects can be minimized by the practitioner choosing the best lens type for an individual patient. Maximizing oxygen transmissibility will limit hypoxic effects, and frequent lens replacement is an effective way of management of deposits.

Success can be enhanced by careful case selection and patient education. Table 12.5 suggests the prerequisites for successful therapeutic lens fitting. Managing patient expectations will also contribute to the overall outcome. These expectations can vary according to the nature of their symptoms. In those patients experiencing acute and recurrent pain (for example, recurrent epithelial erosion), the onset of symptoms is sudden – a seemingly insignificant episode of minor trauma affecting a previously healthy eye. Consequently, they often have high expectations of a simple instant cure.

Careful case selection
Ocular pathology
Adequate patient hygiene
Easy access to clinics
Clearly defined objectives
Therapeutic lenses of varying materials
Water content
Parameters
Adjunctive drug therapy
Clearly defined management strategies
Review procedures
Shared management

Table 12.5
Prerequisites for successful therapeutic lens fitting, adapted from Jackson et al.[2]

In these circumstances, practitioners should explain that while a therapeutic lens can often provide immediate comfort, the underlying cause can take much longer to resolve. Recurrent episodes of pain are common, and lens loss or displacement requires urgent rectification.

In contrast to this group, those with chronic pain, (for example, in bullous keratopathy) are generally aware that they have an ocular pathology which is difficult to treat and hence have more realistic expectations. Although this type of patient may prove easier to manage, the practitioner needs to remain vigilant to stressing the need for urgent action if a problem arises.

Clear instruction on how to seek immediate professional advice if a problem is experienced, both in and out of normal practice hours, should be provided. Prompt action will limit the development of more serious sequelae, or at least reduce the severity of the keratitis. Patients should also be instructed to maintain high standards of personal hygiene, both ocular and general. Lid hygiene procedures should be explained and demonstrated, and for those patients wearing therapeutic lenses on a daily wear basis the importance of hand washing, prior to touching the eye or lenses should be reviewed at each aftercare visit.

Routine instruction on how to insert and remove therapeutic lenses is rarely practical or indicated.

For all therapeutic lens wearers, it is vitally important the practitioner ensures the patient is well instructed on both the need for good hygiene and what action to take if a problem arises. It may also be of benefit to explain to a relative or carer the important signs and symptoms that should be observed. Continued education at each aftercare visit reinforces the importance of the need for urgent action, especially with elderly patients, as they will almost inevitably find the effort and inconvenience of keeping an appointment even greater.

Summary

While therapeutic contact lens fitting is not a part of mainstream practice, practitioners should be familiar with its practice and the techniques involved to enable them to provide advice and appropriate levels of aftercare. In therapeutic lens practice, the objective is rarely to achieve an optimal visual result, rather to protect or assist in the healing process of the compromised cornea.

Almost by definition the eye being fitted with a therapeutic lens is rarely one that is suitable for contact lens wear in the normal sense of that definition. Despite this, the same high level of care must be taken in all aspects of the contact lens fitting and aftercare process. Close collaboration with the medical management of the condition is required, and the practitioner may well need the assistance of people other than the patient to achieve a successful result.

Therapeutic contact lens practice can be rewarding as it can lead to dramatic improvements for the patient in reducing discomfort and aiding the healing process.

Key points
• Therapeutic contact lens practice is a specialist form of practice which should not be undertaken without medical supervision.
• All contact lens practitioners should be aware of the basic aspects of therapeutic lens practice so that they can manage patients in everyday situations and provide support and advice.
• Therapeutic contact lens practice involves achieving the balance between the healing or relieving process and the invasive nature of the contact lens. Correction of visual acuity is rarely the major goal.
• Patient education is as essential in therapeutic lens practice as it is in all forms of contact lens fitting. The education may often have to include other members of the patient's family and additional paramedical staff.

Question 12.1

Which of the following is generally not a primary function of therapeutic lenses?

A Pain relief

B Correcting ametropia

C Promoting epithelial healing

D Sealing corneal perforations

E Improving visual acuity in distorted corneas

Question 12.2

Rigid contact lenses are useful in therapeutic lens fitting because they:

A Are more comfortable

B Allow greater tear exchange

C Are fitted with smaller total diameters

D Form a liquid tear lens and smooth refracting surface

E Have higher oxygen transmissibility

Question 12.3

Which of the following is not an indication for therapeutic lens wear?

A Bullous keratopathy

B Filamentary keratitis

C Meibomian gland dysfunction

D Exposure keratitis

E Recurrent erosion

Question 12.4

Which lens type would be least appropriate for management of exposure keratitis?

A Rigid gas-permeable

B Scleral

C Hydrogel

D Silicone rubber

E Silicone hydrogel

Question 12.5

Potential toxicity effects can be minimized while topical medication is being used concurrently with soft lenses by using:

A Preserved drops

B Daily disposable lenses

C High-water content materials

D Smaller diameter lenses

E Thinner lens designs

Question 12.6

Which of the following is not a prerequisite for successful therapeutic lens fitting?

A Individual practitioner management

B Easy access to clinics

C Careful case selection

D Realistic patient expectations

E Adequate patient selection

Question 12.7

Soft 'bandage lenses' used in therapeutic lens fitting can vary in total diameter from:

A 14.0 mm to 15.0 mm

B 9.0 mm to 12.0 mm

C 14.0 mm to 20.0 mm

D 8.0 mm to 11.0 mm

E 13.0 mm to 15.0 mm

Question 12.8

Which of the following is a less critical requirement of a soft therapeutic lens?

A High oxygen transmissibility

B Choice of total diameters

C Parameter stability

D Large power range

E Economical

Question 12.9

During aftercare of an extended wear bandage lens fit, which of the following may not be necessary?

A Assessment of lens fit

B Visual acuity measurement

C Slit-lamp examination

D Assessment of tissue healing

E Lens removal

Question 12.10

When using rose bengal stain, which of the following statements is false?

A Can result in significant discomfort for the patient

B Can stain lids and skin surrounding the eye

C Tissue staining is best observed under blue light

D Stains dead tissue red

E The tiniest amount possible should be instilled

References

1 Hayworth, N.A.S. and Asbell, P.A. (1990) Therapeutic contact lenses. *CLAO Journal* **16:2** 137–140.

2 Jackson, J. (1996) Therapeutic contact lenses and their use in the management of anterior segment pathology. *JBCLA* **19:1** 11–19.

3 Rubinstein, M.P. (1995) Disposable contact lenses as therapeutic devices. *JBCLA* **18:3** 95–97.

4 John, T., Mobilia, E.F. and Kenyon, K.R. Therapeutic soft contact lenses. In: Ruben, M., Guillon, M. eds. *Contact Lens Practice*. Chapman & Hall Medical 889–912.

5 Weiner, B.M. (1994) Therapeutic bandage lenses. In: Silbert, J.A., ed. *Anterior Segment Complications of Contact Lens Wear*. Churchill Livingstone, 455–471.

6 Pullum, K.W. and Buckley, R.J. (1997) A Study of 530 Px referred for RGP Scleral CL Assessment. *Cornea* **16:6** 612–622.

Answers to multiple choice questions

Question 1.1
Which of the following parts of, or attachments to, the slit-lamp may be used to make objective measurements?
- A Wratten blue filter
- B Graticule
- C Focusing rod
- D Neutral density fitter
- E Joystick movement

Answer B
The graticule allows an objective measurement of anterior features, such as lesions, the horizontal visible iris diameter and pupil size. The other attachments rely upon a practitioner making a qualitative rather than a quantitative assessment.

Question 1.2
Which of the following questions is the preferred means of getting initial background information about a patient's general health?
- A Is your general health good?
- B Are you on any tablets or medication?
- C Tell me about your general health.
- D Do you have any health problems?
- E Are you currently receiving treatment from a doctor?

Answer C
This is the only open question and is most likely to encourage the patient to reveal relevant information. The other options are closed questions and so are more likely to elicit simple 'yes' or 'no' responses. The only caution is with very inhibited or nervous patients when a closed question technique may be the only method to resort to when information is not forthcoming.

Question 1.3
Which of the following reasons explains a cause of contact lens problems in VDU operators?
- A UV radiation from the screen
- B IR radiation from the screen
- C Static field from the screen
- D Reduced blink rate
- E Reduced tear production

Answer D
It has been found that the blink rate reduces during VDU operation potentially leading to inferior corneal desiccation. This should be borne in mind when discussing a patient's occupation and appropriate advice with regard to humidity and blinking should be given.

Question 1.4
In terms of corneal sensitivity, which of the following eye types would you expect to have most problems adapting to hard contact lens wear?
- A Blue irides
- B Aphakics
- C Brown irides
- D Hyperopes
- E Presbyopes

Answer A
Blue-eyed and fair-skinned patients are more likely to have increased corneal sensitivity, as well as a possible increased risk of atopy, and as such are likely to experience greater initial discomfort with rigid lenses.

Question 1.5
Which of the following does NOT occur in the ageing eye?
- A Decreased pupil diameter
- B Reduction in corneal fragility
- C Decreased tonus of lower lid
- D Increased corneal sensitivity
- E Reduced tear stability

Answer D
There is a decrease in corneal sensitivity with age.

Question 1.6
Which of the following general health conditions and associated treatments can influence contact lens wear?
- A Diabetes
- B Systemic hypertension
- C Eczema
- D Thyroid dysfunction
- E All of the above

Answer E
In theory all of the listed conditions can affect contact lens wear. Diabetics may have a more fragile cornea and a reduced corneal sensitivity. Hypertensives may be using medication, which could lead to a dry eye. Eczema is an expression of atopy, which could be associated with deposition and inflammatory responses. Thyroid dysfunction may lead to tear problems and possibly corneal complications due to exposure.

Question 1.7
Which of the following is closest to the ocular refraction of a patient whose spectacle refraction is $-6.00/-2.25 \times 180$?
- A $-5.50/-2.25 \times 180$
- B $-6.00/-2.00 \times 180$
- C $-5.50/-2.00 \times 180$
- D $-6.50/-2.50 \times 180$
- E $-5.75/-2.00 \times 180$

Answer A
Assuming a typical spectacle back vertex distance, one would expect a reduced negative sphere, as one moves closer to the eye, while the amount of astigmatism is maintained.

Question 1.8
A potential contact lens patient presents with meibomian gland dysfunction (MGD) and a pinguecula. Which of the following management options is advised?
- A Refer for surgery for pinguecula and medication for the MGD before fitting
- B Fit without treatment
- C Fit thin soft lenses once MGD has been treated
- D Do not fit lenses
- E Fit large diameter RGP contact lenses

Answer C
The meibomian gland dysfunction may benefit from hot compresses and, once subsided, a fit may be undertaken ensuring minimum mechanical aggravation of the pinguecula. Pingueculae rarely, if ever, require surgical intervention, but may

aggravate poor tear flow, as may occur with long term RGP wear.

Question 1.9
Which of the following statements is false about keratometry?
A Keratometry is a good indication of hard lens base curve selection
B Keratometry is a good indication of soft lens base curve selection
C The keratometer can be used to assess tear quantity
D Keratometry measures the central of cornea
E Keratometry measurements can be recorded in mm and/or dioptres

Answer C
Keratometry measures the central corneal curvature over an area of approximately 3 to 6 mm. It records the value in dioptres or mm. The reflection of the mires gives some qualitative information about the tears but little of the actual quantity.

Question 1.10
What is the preferred method for measuring the size of a corneal lesion?
A Hand-held mm rule
B Grading scale
C Slit-lamp eyepiece graticule
D Slit-lamp beam width/height adjustment
E Keratometer

Answer C
A slit-lamp eyepiece graticule is the preferred method of measuring anterior lesions with some degree of accuracy.

Question 2.1
In which of the following does the biomicroscope not play a role?
A Assessing corneal shape factor
B Assessing hard lens fitting characteristics
C Evaluating neovascularization
D Judging extent of lens deposits
E Assessing soft lens fitting characteristics

Answer A
Corneal shape factor and topographic detail are best established by keratometry and topographical instrumentation.

Question 2.2
Which of the following statements about the slit-lamp is true?

A The red free enhances the contrast of corneal staining
B The illumination and observation systems are coupled to maximize light intensity on the cornea
C A photo-slit lamp is essential if the practitioner wants to photograph the eye
D The illumination and observation systems are coupled to allow a three dimensional view of the eye
E None of the above

Answer E
The red free filter is best to enhance contrast of red structures, such as new vessels. Coupling of the illumination and viewing systems allow the observer to view illuminated areas from a different viewpoint so allowing cross-sectional observation. Illumination is maximized with a rheostat and three-dimensional viewing is allowed by a binocular viewing system. Though a photo slit-lamp is useful, there are other methods of photographing or imaging the eye. Therefore none of the options given are strictly true.

Question 2.3
Which of the following is best visualized using high magnification direct illumination with a narrow slit beam?
A Neovascularization
B Striae
C Microcysts
D Corneal staining
E All of the above

Answer B
Striae are best seen at high magnification directly with a narrow beam. Microcysts show up better in indirect illumination, neovascularization with a wider beam and staining at a magnification dictated by its extent.

Question 2.4
Which of the following is best viewed using high magnification, indirect illumination and a narrow slit beam?
A Endothelial folds
B Microcysts
C Polymegathism
D Depth of corneal lesions
E Dellen

Answer B
Microcysts are best evaluated under indirect illumination.

Question 2.5
Which of the following should be recorded as a subjective grade?
A Microcysts
B Palpebral hyperaemia
C Endothelial folds
D Size of corneal opacities
E Neovascularization

Answer B
Hyperaemia in general is difficult to either count or measure so is best noted in terms of a grading system.

Question 2.6
Why is a yellow barrier filter recommended?
A To be placed over the illumination system to enhance contrast when using fluorescein
B To be placed over the observation system to enhance contrast when using fluorescein
C To shift the wavelength of the incident light on the cornea
D To help in assessment of neovascularization
E To filter out reflected light of 520 nm

Answer B
Placing a yellow filter over the observation system allows some absorption of the reflected blue light from the cobalt filter so increasing the contrast of the fluorescein pattern.

Question 2.7
Using the FDA grading scale, how would the SEAL in Figure 2.11(d) be graded?
A 0
B 1
C 2
D 3
E 4

Answer C
The image is one of a moderate SEAL change that may well require clinical intervention.

Question 2.8
When should fluorescein be used?
A At the preliminary examination and rigid lens aftercare
B At the initial examination and all lens aftercare
C At the initial examination and when a problem is suspected with soft lenses
D Only with rigid lens wearers

E Only in symptomatic contact lens wearers

Answer B
Fluorescein assessment is essential at all visits of the contact lens patient.

Question 2.9
How can contact lens deposits best be viewed with the slit-lamp?
A *In vivo*, direct illumination high magnification
B *In vivo*, indirect illumination high magnification
C By sclerotic scatter
D *In vitro* using diffuse illumination
E *In vitro* using an optic section

Answer D
Deposits are best viewed in a dark room, the lens removed from the patient. Diffuse illumination prevents single reflections from masking any areas of deposition.

Question 2.10
Which of the following statements concerning lid eversion is false?
A Carry out with fluorescein instilled
B Permits detection of CLPC
C Carry out prior to tear film assessment
D Forms part of routine aftercare for all contact lens wearers
E Forms part of preliminary examination

Answer C
Lid eversion may affect the integrity of the tear film and so should be carried out after an in-depth tear assessment.

Question 3.1
Which of the following can the keratometer not be used for?
A Judging the fit of a soft contact lens
B Choosing the base curve of a RGP lens
C Measuring a corneal curvature
D Assessing tear film quality
E Measuring lenticular astigmatism

Answer A
The fit of a soft lens is best viewed with a slit-lamp biomicroscope. The keratometer, while giving useful information about the quality and shape of the reflecting surface, has limited use here.

Question 3.2
Which of the following instruments can provide immediate information about corneal shape factor?
A Placido disc
B One-position keratometer
C Photokeratoscope
D Two-position keratometer
E Variable doubling keratoscopy

Answer C
The shape factor is an indication of the variation in curvature across the surface of the cornea and traditional keratometers do not measure this. While a placido disc will give qualitative information about the variable curvature, a photokeratoscope gives immediate access to this information quantitatively.

Question 3.3
Modern computerized videokeratoscopes typically analyse what number of data points?
A Two
B 3.2
C 6 000
D 14 000
E 140 000

Answer D
Typically 14 000 data points are analysed with modern computerized videokeratoscopes.

Question 3.4
Which of the following statements about the cornea is true?
A The cornea is like an oblate ellipse, steepening towards the periphery
B The cornea is like an oblate ellipse, flattening towards the periphery
C The cornea is like a prolate ellipse, steepening towards the periphery
D The cornea is like a prolate ellipse, flattening towards the periphery
E The cornea is like an oblate sphere, steepening towards the periphery

Answer B
The cornea is likened to an oblate ellipse which flattens gradually towards its periphery.

Question 3.5
Which of the following should the practitioner do before measuring corneal radius with the keratometer?
A Focus the instrument mires on the cornea

B Set the objective to the patient's refractive error
C Ensure the eyepiece is focused against a white background
D Ensure that the patient's accommodation is relaxed
E Check that the doubling device is zeroed

Answer C
Before a measurement is taken, the practitioner should focus the eyepiece against a white background. If the eyepiece is not in focus then any readings obtained will not be accurate.

Question 3.6
Which of the following statements is true in variable doubling?
A The distance between the object and the image is varied
B The object size remains constant
C The image size remains constant
D The distance between the mires is varied
E The subject observes multiple targets

Answer B
In variable doubling keratometry, the object size remains constant. This is why this form of instrument is useful in assessing tear break-up in a non-invasive manner.

Question 3.7
How could the practitioner measure the K-readings of an advanced keratoconic patient whose readings were off the scale?
A Add a +1.25DS lens in front of the keratometer objective
B Add a +2.75DS lens in front of the keratometer objective
C Add a +0.75DS lens in front of the keratometer objective
D Add a −1.25DS lens in front of the keratometer objective
E Add a −1.75DS lens in front of the keratometer objective

Answer A
If the cornea is excessively steep, as with an advanced keratoconic, a +1.25D lens may be used in conjunction with the instrument, provided recalibration is carried out. Negative lenses are needed for excessively flattened corneas.

Question 3.8
How can the peripheral corneal radius be measured?

A   Using the placido disc
B   Focusing the keratometer on the limbus
C   Taking measurements with the eye in different positions
D   Add a +0.75DS lens in front of the keratometer objective
E   Uncoupling the doubling system

Answer C
The patient may be asked to fixate upon four targets around the object, so allowing peripheral measurements to be taken. This is often far from ideal, however, due to inter-patient variation in anatomy and the stability of fixation.

Question 3.9
What is the basis of keratoscopy?
A   Peripheral keratometry readings with a moving objective
B   The placido disc
C   Laser interference assessment
D   Confocal laser measurement
E   Multiple doubling systems

Answer B
The placido disc is a simple concentric ring target which will give an immediate indication of curvature variation which may be analysed and quantified subsequently. This forms the basis of photokeratoscopy.

Question 3.10
What is the mean shape factor for the steep meridian of caucasian eyes?
A   0
B   0.5
C   0.81
D   0.83
E   1

Answer C
The corneal shape factor of the Caucasian eye has a mean value of 0.83 for the flat meridian and 0.81 for the steep meridian.

Question 4.1
The tear compound which enables the tears to wet the normal epithelium is:
A   Secreted from the meibomian glands
B   A glycoprotein layer on the anterior surface of the tears
C   Produced from the glands of Moll and Krause
D   An ester wax
E   Provides an optically smooth surface

Answer C
The mucus layer of the tear film renders the corneal epithelium hydrophilic to enhance wetting by the aqueous layer. This is possible due to secretion from the glands of Moll and Krause together with the activity of conjunctival goblet cells.

Question 4.2
The stimulus for blinking and replenishment of the tear film is:
A   Excess lipid distribution in the inferior fornix
B   Loss of hydrophilicity of the mucus contaminated by lipid
C   Excess mucus accumulation in the inferior fornix
D   Evaporation of the surface lipid layer
E   Contamination of the lipid layer with glycoproteins

Answer B
As the tear film reduces due to evaporation, there is a diffusion of lipid towards the mucus layer. As mucus is contaminated by lipid, the tear film ruptures and isolated areas of break-up occur so stimulating the next blink.

Question 4.3
The tear film of an RGP wearer:
A   Has a decreased NIBUT in comparison to a non-wearer
B   Has a thicker lipid layer than a non-wearer
C   Has a more stable lipid layer than a non-contact lens wearer
D   Contains no mucus layer
E   Maintains its stability through producing more aqueous layer

Answer A
It is difficult for the tear film to maintain a lipid layer over the RGP lens as seen by the reduced non-invasive tear break-up time (NIBUT) of an RGP wearer compared to that of a non-lens wearer.

Question 4.4
The tear film of a soft lens wearer is not influenced by:
A   Water content
B   Lens movement
C   Lens thickness
D   Ocular lubricant
E   Lens deposition

Answer D
Ocular lubricants are used to resolve the problem of dry eye in soft contact lens wearers, but no one has yet shown any significant lasting effect upon the nature of the tear film.

Question 4.5
Which of the following provides an assessment of tear quantity?
A   HIR-CAL grid
B   Assessment of keratometry image
C   Inferior tear prism height
D   Loveridge grid
E   Specular reflection

Answer C
While the other options give useful information about the tear quality, the inferior tear prism height is a useful guide to the tear volume. As such, the authors advocate its use as an integral part of the preassessment of potential contact lens wearers.

Question 4.6
Which of the following is true?
A   The Loveridge grid fits on to the keratometer and assesses tear quality
B   The Tearscope provides a means of assessing tear production
C   NIBUT values obtained with the HIR-CAL are greater than those found with fluorescein
D   NIBUT values obtained with the HIR-CAL are less than those found with fluorescein
E   The HIR-CAL grid can also be used for assessing corneal radius

Answer C
The HIR-CAL grid provides a non-invasive assessment of tear break-up time (NIBUT) and as such may give readings of up to 30 seconds longer than fluorescein BUT measurements.

Question 4.7
Which of the following tear patterns is most likely to be associated with contact lens drying problems?
A   Closed marmoreal
B   Stable amorphous
C   Open marmoreal
D   Trace colour fringes
E   Flow

Answer C
Closed marmoreal, stable amorphous and flow patterns are all representative of stable tear films. Trace colour fringes may indicate

some excess lipid deposition potential but contact lens wear is likely to be acceptable. An open marmoreal pattern, however, would be expected to give contact lens drying problems.

Question 4.8
Which of the following statements about the Tearscope is FALSE?
A   Is the only way to visualize the relative thickness of the tear film
B   Should be used with a biomicroscope
C   Provides an assessment of NIBUT
D   Assesses tear quality
E   Allows assessment of the lipid layer

Answer A
The Tearscope allows measurement of the non-invasive tear break-up time and assessment of the lipid layer. It would not be useful for tear film thickness measurement.

Question 4.9
What is the major advantage of measuring NIBUT?
A   It can be carried out at the same time as keratometry
B   It gives information about tear quality, as well as quantity
C   It assesses a larger area of the tear film
D   The tear film is examined in a more natural state
E   Tear film evaporation is minimal

Answer D
It might be strongly argued that the use of fluorescein allows a measure of the break-up time of the tear film when it has fluorescein in it. A non-invasive technique is more akin to that of the tear film in its natural state so is preferable.

Question 4.10
Compared to pre-ocular tear film, the pre-lens tear film is:
A   Thicker
B   More stable
C   Same thickness
D   Thinner
E   More easily observed

Answer D
The pre-lens tear film is thinner and less stable than the pre-ocular tear film.

Question 5.1
Which of the following characteristics should a well fitting soft lens NOT show?

A   Corneal coverage in all positions of gaze
B   1 mm post blink movement
C   Smooth return on push-up test
D   Edge alignment to the conjunctiva
E   High level of patient comfort and vision

Answer B
It is known that movement of a soft lens plays little part in corneal oxygenation and movement of 1 mm on blinking would only serve to increase patient awareness of the lens. Good corneal coverage is essential to avoid desiccation of the cornea. Smooth return on push-up and edge alignment are both characteristic of a good fit and should lead to a high level of patient comfort and vision.

Question 5.2
Central keratometry readings:
A   Predict the BOZR to be chosen for a trial soft lens
B   Provide baseline data of corneal contour
C   Provide a means of judging tear quantity
D   Correlate with the total sag of the best fitting soft lens
E   Measure degree of peripheral corneal flattening

Answer B
Keratometry is a poor indicator of soft lens fit. However, the technique may still be useful as the other options still hold true.

Question 5.3
When inserting a soft trial lens, symptoms of initial discomfort cannot be caused by:
A   Differences between tear pH and the pH of the storage solutions
B   Excessive lens movement caused by a loose lens and reflex tearing
C   Differences between osmolarity of tears and storage solutions
D   Insufficient lens movement
E   Excessive edge stand-off from the conjunctiva

Answer D
A lens with insufficient movement would lead to less discomfort, as there would be less mechanical compromise of adjoining tissue. It is quite possible for a very tight, immovable lens to still feel quite comfortable.

Question 5.4
The following assessments should NOT be

made while viewing with the slit-lamp:
A   Corneal centration
B   Post-blink movement
C   Visual stability
D   Recovery following push-up test
E   Conjunctival alignment

Answer C
Though the other four options which may be assessed at the slit-lamp may well influence visual stability, it is not useful to assess the status of vision at the slit-lamp.

Question 5.5
Squeeze pressure:
A   Is directly correlated with post-blink movement
B   Is an assessment of the oxygen flux benefits
C   Has a decreasing exponential relationship with lens tightness
D   Is a valuable means of assessing conjunctival alignment
E   Has a linear relationship with lens tightness as measured by push-up test

Answer E
As illustrated by the figure in the text, tightness as shown by the push-up test has a linear relationship with squeeze pressure and so should be considered the arbitrator in judging lens fit.

Question 5.6
Which of the following external factors will not have an influence on lens fit?
A   Corneal thickness
B   Tear pH
C   Corneal apex position
D   Lid pressure
E   Ocular sag

Answer A
Corneal thickness will not influence lens fit. A reduced pH may lead to lens steepening. A displaced corneal apex will lead to a decentred lens. Increased lid pressure, as with tight lids, may lead to excessive movement. If the ocular sag is less than the lens sag then a tight fit is likely.

Question 5.7
Which of the following lens factors will not have an influence on lens fit?
A   Peripheral lens design
B   Water content of material
C   Lens sagittal depth
D   Lens total diameter

E   Handling tint

Answer E
The handling tint will have no influence upon the lens fit. All the other options will.

Question 5.8
If a lens decentres, which of the following strategies could the practitioner use to improve the centration?
A   Increase BOZR, maintain same TD
B   Decrease BOZR, maintain same TD
C   Increase BOZR, increase TD
D   Increase lens thickness
E   Decrease TD, maintain BOZR

Answer B
A steeper fit would reduce the likelihood of lens decentration, and hence a reduced BOZR would allow this. Steepening might also be achieved by increasing the TD which serves to expand the sag of the lens.

Question 5.9
If a trial lens shows no significant post-blink movement, the practitioner should first:
A   Use the push-up test to determine whether the fit is satisfactory
B   Increase the BOZR
C   Increase the water content of the lens
D   Decrease the thickness of the lens
E   Decrease the TD

Answer A
Though there may be no observable post-blink movement, a push-up test is essential to verify that this is indeed due to a tight fit. If confirmed, then the lens parameters may be adjusted to flatten the fit.

Question 5.10
Which of the following will have the greatest impact on loosening a lens fit?
A   Flatten BOZR, increase TD
B   Steeper BOZR, reduce TD
C   Flatten BOZR, reduce TD
D   Steeper BOZR, increase TD
E   Flatten BOZR only

Answer C
Both lengthening or flattening the BOZR and reducing the TD will serve to loosen a lens fit.

Question 6.1
A well fitting RGP lens should ideally show:
A   Full corneal coverage in all positions of gaze
B   No vertical post-blink movement

C   Pupil coverage by the BOZD
D   Central apical corneal contact
E   No edge clearance

Answer C
If the BOZD fails to cover the pupil adequately then the patient may well suffer from the scatter of light from the peripheral curves and experience flare.

Question 6.2
A difference of 0.4 mm between steepest and flattest keratometry readings equates approximately to:
A   4.00D of corneal astigmatism
B   1.00D of lenticular astigmatism
C   2.00D of corneal astigmatism
D   1.00D of corneal astigmatism
E   2.00D of lenticular astigmatism

Answer C
0.1 mm on the keratometer equates to 0.5D of corneal astigmatism, hence 0.4 mm will equate to 2.00D of corneal astigmatism.

Question 6.3
In which of the following prescriptions will a spherical RGP lens not provide satisfactory vision?
A   Rx: -2.00 DS
    K: 7.60 al 180 - 7.60 al 90
B   Rx: -2.00 DS/-2.00DC × 180
    K: 7.60 al 180 - 7.20 al 90
C   Rx: -2.00 DS/-2.00DC × 180
    K: 7.60 al 180 - 7.50 al 90
D   Rx: -5.00/+2.00 × 180
    K: 8.00 al 90 - 7.60 al 180
E   Rx: −3.00/−2.00 × 90
    K: 7.60 al 180 - 8.00 al 90

Answer C
In this instance there is 2.00D of cylinder in the spectacle refraction while the K-readings indicate that only 0.5D of this is corneal. The remaining 1.50D is likely to be lenticular and this would remain uncorrected if a spherical RGP lens is fitted. This would therefore leave the patient blurred by this amount.

Question 6.4
Which of the following will over-refraction not give information about:
A   Alignment of back surface of lens to cornea
B   Flexure of lens
C   Required lens power
D   Degree of corneal eccentricity
E   Tear lens thickness

Answer D
As well as giving information relating to the required lens power, including the influence of the tear lens, over-refraction gives some indication of the flexure of the lens. It will not, however, give any indication of corneal eccentricity.

Question 6.5
A patient has K-readings of 7.80 al 180 and 7.40 al 90. Which spherical back surface lens should be the trial lens of first choice?
A   7.40
B   7.20
C   7.90
D   7.70
E   7.60

Answer D
This patient has 2.00D of corneal astigmatism. For smaller amounts of cylinder, a practitioner may fit upon the flattest K-reading. For this degree of astigmatism, a lens that is 0.05 to 0.1 steeper than the flattest K-reading is appropriate to minimize flexure and to maintain stable acuity.

Question 6.6
A patient complains of poor comfort while wearing an RGP lens. This is unlikely to be caused by:
A   Excess lens movement
B   Trapped foreign body
C   Excess edge clearance
D   Lenticular astigmatism
E   Poor wetting

Answer D
Though lenticular astigmatism may affect the clarity of vision, it will not have any impact upon comfort. All other options may lead to discomfort.

Question 6.7
Which of the following is unlikely to be a cause of poor vision in an RGP lens wearer?
A   Lens flexure
B   Excess edge clearance
C   Poor wetting
D   Residual astigmatism
E   Change in corneal shape

Answer B
Excessive edge clearance would decrease comfort and perhaps lead to variable vision indirectly due to a tearing response, but it does not directly reduce vision.

Question 6.8
A patient experiences 'flare' resulting from an RGP lens that rides high and does not drop with the blink. Which of the following statements is true?
  A The patient probably has against the rule astigmatism
  B The lens probably needs a larger TD and BOZD
  C The patient may require a toric front surface design
  D The lens probably requires cleaning and polishing
  E The lens material probably needs changing

Answer B
The lens is positioned such that there is light scatter from the peripheral curves and so a larger BOZD and TD would aid the centration and prevent the flare.

Question 6.9
Which of the following would not cause decentration of an RGP lens?
  A Displaced corneal apex
  B Against the rule astigmatism
  C Excessive lacrimation
  D Total diameter too small
  E Total diameter too large

Answer E
As with the previous question, the larger diameter would aid centration, the other options are all capable of promoting decentration.

Question 6.10
Which of the following lenses should be chosen to achieve the same optical corrections as a lens with a BOZR of 7.80 and a power of +3.00?
  A 7.90 + 3.50
  B 7.90 + 2.50
  C 7.90 + 3.25
  D 7.90 + 2.75
  E 7.85 + 3.25

Answer A
The lens is flatter by 0.10 mm which would give a negative tear lens of -0.50 so negating the extra +0.50D of the contact lens power.

Question 7.1
Approximately what percentage of prescriptions have 0.75DC or more of ocular astigmatism?
  A 20 per cent

  B 10 per cent
  C 16 per cent
  D 33 per cent
  E 5 per cent

Answer D
As much as 33 per cent of refractive errors include astigmatism of 0.75D or more.

Question 7.2
Which of the following cannot be used to correct an astigmatic refractive error in the majority of cases?
  A Aspheric RGP
  B Toric periphery
  C Spherical RGP
  D Bi-toric RGP
  E Spherical soft

Answer E
Spherical soft contact lenses will not correct corneal or lenticular astigmatism, as they will assume the corneal topography. They are useful, however, in the situation where a spherical refractive error is a result of lenticular astigmatism neutralizing corneal astigmatism as they will maintain the refractive element of the cornea.

Question 7.3
What area of a prism-stabilized soft toric lens is the thinnest?
  A Centre
  B Superior
  C Inferior
  D Nasal
  E Temporal

Answer B
The thinning of the superior portion of the lens allows the upper lid to squeeze the thicker inferior portion downwards.

Question 7.4
Which area of a dynamic stabilized soft toric lens is the thinnest?
  A Centre
  B Superior and inferior
  C Inferior
  D Superior
  E Temporal and nasal

Answer B
The thinner superior and inferior areas allow the lids to maintain the thicker lateral regions in the interpalpebral space.

Question 7.5
Successful toric soft lens fitting requires:

  A No lens movement
  B Rotational stability
  C Thinner lens design
  D Smaller TD
  E Excessive lens movement

Answer B
Unstable rotation will not allow for a stable cylinder correction so resulting in variable or poor visual performance.

Question 7.6
Orientation of a soft toric contact lens does not rely on:
  A Lid/lens interaction
  B Lens power
  C Lens thickness profile
  D Gravity
  E Overall fit

Answer D
Gravity has been shown not to play a significant part in stabilizing the lens on the eye.

Question 7.7
Axes of astigmatism less than 2.00DC are distributed:
  A Almost equally around the clock face
  B More commonly 'with the rule'
  C More commonly 'against the rule'
  D More commonly with oblique axes
  E Predominantly associated 'with and against' the rule

Answer A
Despite the somewhat misleading terms 'with the rule' and 'against the rule' when used in a wider context, it has been found that axes for small cylinders are spread almost equally around the clock face.

Question 7.8
Axes of astigmatism greater than 2.50DC are distributed:
  A Almost equally around the clock face
  B More commonly 'with the rule'
  C More commonly 'against the rule'
  D More commonly with oblique axes
  E Predominantly associated 'with and against' the rule

Answer B
As cylinder power increases, the percentage of axes falling in the 'with the rule' category increases. Fifty per cent of the axes for cylinders of 2.50D may be classified in this manner.

Question 7.9

A spectacle refraction is found to be, $-6.00/-2.25 \times 10$ at vertex distance 10 mm. What lens power would you initially trial?

 A $-6.00/-2.25 \times 10$
 B $-5.75/-2.00 \times 10$
 C $-5.50/-2.25 \times 10$
 D $-5.75/-1.75 \times 10$
 E $-5.50/-1.75 \times 10$

Answer E

The reduced sphere and cylinder power reflects the reduction in minus lens power needed the closer one is to the cornea.

Question 7.10

An ocular refraction is found to be $-2.00/-1.75 \times 180°$. A trial lens placed on the eye rotates anticlockwise by $10°$. What lens prescription would you order to compensate for this?

 A $-2.00/-1.75 \times 180°$
 B $-2.00/-1.75 \times 10°$
 C $-2.00/-1.75 \times 170°$
 D $-2.00/-1.75 \times 90°$
 E $-2.00/-1.75 \times 80°$

Answer C

By specifying an axis of $170°$, the anticlockwise rotation of $10°$ will leave the lens orientated at the $180°$ required.

Question 8.1

If a $+2.00$ blur test results in the patient reporting that the image is clearest when the $+2.00$D lens is held in front of the left eye, then:

 A The patient is left eye dominant
 B No strong dominance is present
 C The patient is right eye dominant
 D The patient is left handed
 E The patient is right handed

Answer C

In order for monovision to be acceptable to a patient it is essential for the visual system to suppress the blurred image. The visual system is more successful at suppressing an image within the non-dominant eye so it is important for the practitioner to identify which eye this is in order to decide which lens to place in which eye. By significantly blurring with $+2.00$D either eye, the patient will report clearer or more comfortable vision when the fog is presented before the non-dominant eye. This assumes distance dominance, the patient being asked to view a distance target.

Question 8.2

Which of the following is NOT an advantage of monovision?

 A Good near vision performance
 B Success rates at least equal to bifocal lens fitting
 C Easy to trial
 D Full stereopsis
 E Full choice of lens design and material type

Answer D

The reduction in clarity of one of the two images from the eyes will lead to a reduced stereopsis and this might be expressed as a reduced ability to judge distances or depths.

Question 8.3

Which of the following statements regarding alternating bifocal lenses is FALSE?

 A Fused and solid designs are available
 B Are usually fitted steeper than flattest K
 C Visual quality is high with successful fits
 D Prism is used to control lens stability and position
 E Lower eyelid tone is important to enable adequate lens translation

Answer B

A steeper fit would reduce the mobility of the lens on the eye. For the alternating bifocal design of contact lens to work, it is important for the lens to be mobile so that, upon looking at a near object, the lower lid will raise the lens and allow light to enter the pupil via the near segment. A flatter fit will therefore encourage lens mobility.

Question 8.4

Which of the following statements is FALSE in relation to simultaneous vision lens fitting?

 A Lens centration is important
 B 0.25D adjustments can have a profound effect on visual performance
 C Over-refraction using a phoropter is preferred
 D Objective vision measurement alone is not a good predictor of success
 E Modified and enhanced monovision fitting techniques can be explored when necessary

Answer C

The simultaneous lens design relies upon the focusing of two retinal images corres-

ponding to distance and near targets. This is achieved in a number of ways but all of them rely upon a change in the refractive properties of the lens from its centre to the periphery. This therefore makes this design of lens very much pupil-dependent, as a small pupil will tend to minimize the input of light rays through more peripheral areas of the lens. Use of a phoropter will decrease the amount of light upon an eye and tend to encourage a mydriasis. This will then mean that the focusing properties of the lens are being assessed in conditions other than those in which the lens is normally worn.

Question 8.5

Back-surface aspheric soft lens designs are usually:

 A Centre-near type designs
 B Distance image bias in high luminance lighting levels
 C Distance image bias in low luminance lighting levels
 D Designed to correct greater than 1.50D of presbyopia
 E Near image bias in low luminance lighting levels

Answer B

The back surface asphericity allows for a peripheral flattening of the lens, the rate of which dictates the degree of difference in focusing from the centre of the lens to the periphery. In high luminance levels (or indeed upon looking at near objects), the pupil will constrict and this will tend to favour light passing through the centre of the lens and hence give a distance bias.

Question 8.6

Modified monovision fitting approach involves:

 A Reducing the add power during monovision fitting
 B Fitting one eye with a single-vision lens and the other with a bifocal
 C Ensuring both eyes are fitted with alternative centre-near designs
 D Fitting a translating lens design in one eye and a simultaneous lens design in the other
 E Altering distance or near power to enhance distance vision in one eye and near in the other

Answer E

As opposed to enhanced monovision, where a single vision lens is placed before one, usually the dominant, eye and a bifocal before the other, modified monovision is now generally used to describe the use of two bifocal lenses. One of the bifocal lenses is biased towards the distance while the other is near-biased. Those patients who find the clarity binocularly of the original non-modified lens intolerable or unsatisfactory prefer this. For this technique to be successful, it is necessary to have information about ocular dominance and binocular state, just as in 'true' monovision.

The modified monovision may be achieved in a variety of ways including a straightforward adjustment of the refractive power of a lens, to using combinations of alternating design to bias one lens to distance and the other to near.

Question 8.7
The percentage of UK presbyopic patients over the age of 45 is:
A   16 per cent
B   31 per cent
C   47 per cent
D   28 per cent
E   64 per cent

Answer C
UK demographic figures suggest that 47 per cent of the population are over 45 years of age and thus experience presbyopia.

Question 8.8
Which of the following statements is TRUE about multi-zone concentric bifocal designs?
A   Allow distance and near vision by lens translation
B   Enhance near image contrast in high luminance lighting
C   Consist of two distance powered zones and one near
D   Minimize the dependency of lens function on pupil size
E   Enhance near image contrast in low luminance lighting levels

Answer D
Multi-zone lenses were introduced as a way of reducing the dependency of presbyopic lenses upon pupil size. Alternating the near and distance zones concentrically helps reduce the effects of pupil size change.

Question 8.9
When fitting alternating vision bifocals, the segment top position during primary gaze should be approximately:
A   Midway between lower pupil margin and inferior limbus
B   In line with the lower pupil margin
C   Bisecting the pupil horizontally
D   In line with the upper pupil margin
E   Midway between upper pupil margin and superior limbus

Answer B
By placing the segment top in line with the lower pupil margin in the primary gaze position, the lens will move up upon downgaze and the near segment will be over the pupil.

Question 8.10
Which of the following statements is FALSE about simultaneous vision correction?
A   Are available in both soft and rigid materials
B   Rely on the visual system to 'select' the clearer picture
C   Result in less reduction in stereopsis when compared to monovision
D   Result in the same subjective and objective visual performance as a spectacle lens correction
E   Lens adjustments can be made based on knowledge of ocular dominance

Answer D
Simultaneous vision by its very nature presents two images simultaneously and therefore cannot replicate the clarity and degree of contrast of a spectacle lens correction, as will be appreciated when questioning the patient.

Question 9.1
Which lens fitting will subsequently require more frequent initial and ongoing aftercare?
A   Neophyte daily wear new fit
B   Existing daily wear refit to alternative daily wear lens
C   Neophyte extended wear new fit
D   Existing extended wear refit to daily wear modality
E   Existing extended wear refit to alternative extended wear lens

Answer C
A neophyte or new fit will always require closer monitoring during the early stages of wear compared to an experienced existing lens wearer. Many of the possible complications due to inappropriate fitting or intolerance to wear may be exhibited during this initial period. A new extended wear patient should be seen again, after an initial trial period, immediately after the first overnight wear period to establish suitability for the extended wear regime.

Question 9.2
Which of the following clinical observations is more likely to result in patient symptoms?
A   Vascularization
B   Microcysts
C   Low-grade CLPC
D   Infiltrate (no overlying epithelial staining)
E   Diffuse epithelial staining resulting from toxic reaction

Answer E
Although there is always great subjective variation between patients in the reporting of any symptom, there is unlikely to be any symptom reported with neovascularization, microcysts or infiltrates without staining. Low grade CLPC, where papillae have yet to be established significantly, is unlikely to result in either discomfort or blurring from the tear film. Because of the distribution of the corneal nerves, there is an associated discomfort with epithelial compromise and the diffuse stain found as a response to a toxic reaction typically presents with reports of discomfort after a period of wear.

Question 9.3
Which aspects of vision assessment would not be carried out routinely during contact lens aftercare?
A   Visual acuity
B   Stereopsis
C   Oculomotor balance
D   Subjective visual quality
E   Quality of retinoscopy reflex

Answer B
Visual acuity measurement is a legal requirement and should be carried out and recorded before a physical examination of the eye is undertaken. It is also important to remember that Snellen acuity alone may not represent changes in the visual quality a patient may achieve and hence this needs to be ascertained also. With higher refractive errors, the prismatic effects of spectacles may lead to changes in the oculomotor balance which needs to be monitored. Retinoscopy is a useful means of detecting over-refraction requirements as well as giving information about the quality of light transmission through the cornea and contact lens.

Question 9.4
Acute and/or chronic corneal oedema resulting from soft lens wear will not result in which of the following clinical signs?
A Microcysts
B Central corneal clouding
C Vertical striae
D Vascularization
E Epithelial staining

Answer B
Hard non-gas permeable lens wearers may exhibit significant corneal oedema. The small diameter of the lens leads to the main oedematous response falling within a central corneal oedematous zone manifesting itself as central corneal clouding. This is unlikely with a soft lens as the corneal coverage will not localize oedematous response to a central area. Central corneal clouding is usefully visualized using sclerotic scatter in a dark room.

Question 9.5
Which of the following is imperative at every aftercare visit?
A Use of fluorescein during slit-lamp examination
B Keratometry measurements
C Ophthalmoscopy
D Spectacle refraction
E Lid eversion

Answer A
As indicated in Question 3, there are many measurements that should be considered at every aftercare appointment. While lid eversion is important to establish the presence of, and to monitor, any allergic or follicular responses, it goes along with ophthalmoscopy as a part of the practitioner's responsibility in maintaining the integrity of ocular health. Fluorescein assessment is imperative at every visit, however, as it is the best way to assess the state of the cornea and to detect early epithelial changes which may warrant changes in contact lens wear.

Question 9.6
Which of the following signs/symptoms is more typical of a sterile keratitis?
A Central lesion
B Lesion >1 mm
C Uveitis
D Progressive clinical signs
E Mild pain

Answer E
An infective keratitis is more likely to present with progressive and severe pain, alongside other typical symptoms and signs such as central lesions (which may be larger than 1 mm in diameter), epithelial defects, progressive and severe corneal suppuration and an associated uveitis. A sterile keratitis will be unlikely to cause any discomfort worse than mild pain.

Question 9.7
Which of the following statements concerning aftercare appointments is true?
A Patients should decide the frequency of visit
B Aftercares are only needed whenever a patient is suffering any symptoms of discomfort
C The patient should always attend wearing their current contact lenses except in unusual circumstances
D Vision is assessed during routine eye examinations so is not a consideration at an aftercare appointment
E Reminders to patients to attend for aftercare appointments have proven useless

Answer C
It is important for the practitioner to see the lenses *in situ*, preferably after a period of wear. It may also be revealing to see the case for the lenses and often to note the condition of any back-up spectacles. Only when there is the suspicion of a pathological reaction, such as a red eye, should the patient be instructed to remove their lenses before consulting the practitioner.

Question 9.8
Which of the following is most likely to lead to an inferior corneal 'smile' stain?
A Toxic response
B Foreign body beneath the upper lid
C Hypoxic response
D Desiccation with soft lens wear
E Desiccation with RGP lens wear

Answer D
The 'smile' stain is typical of incomplete lid closure, as in lagophthalmos, or in prolonged soft lens wear when the eye is drying. An RGP wearer exhibiting desiccation would typically show 3 and 9 o'clock staining.

Question 9.9
Which of the following statements concerning visual compromise reported at an aftercare appointment is true?
A Deposits would lead to an improved acuity post-blink
B Deposits would lead to a reduced acuity post-blink
C A loose fitting lens would give an improved acuity post-blink
D A lens that was inside out would give an improved post-blink acuity
E Corneal oedema would give an improved post-blink acuity

Answer A
Typically the re-wetting that occurs subsequent to a blink would improve the optical clarity of a deposited lens surface but the deposits would cause a tear film disruption rapidly so degrading the acuity through the lens after some moments, despite an initial improvement.

Question 9.10
Which of the following would typically cause a gradual worsening of acuity as the day progresses?
A Loose-fitting lens
B Flare
C Foreign body
D Corneal oedema
E Inappropriate refractive correction

Answer D
Corneal oedema would take sometimes hours to establish to a level that would cause a subjective reduction in visual quality for the wearer.

Question 10.1
Which of the following ocular conditions would not be due to a solution reaction?
A Diffuse corneal staining
B Corneal ulceration
C Conjunctival staining
D Conjunctival hyperaemia
E Tarsal palpebral hyperaemia and follicles

Answer B
Corneal ulceration is a significant finding that may be due to contact lens wear or an inflammatory response to localized corneal compromise but would not result from solutions.

Question 10.2
Which of the following statements regard-

ing 3% hydrogen peroxide is false?
- A Hydrogen peroxide is an effective bactericidal agent
- B Hydrogen peroxide can be broken down into oxygen and water
- C Hydrogen peroxide can cause changes to soft lens parameters
- D Hydrogen peroxide does not need neutralizing before lens insertion
- E Hydrogen peroxide systems are generally free from preservatives

Answer D

Hydrogen peroxide in a concentration of 3% must always be neutralized before coming in contact with the eye otherwise significant discomfort will result, something many contact lens wearers will testify to!

Question 10.3

Poor comfort on lens insertion could not be due to?
- A Residual peroxide on lens
- B Non-wetted lens
- C Tonicity imbalance with tear film
- D Residual cleaning solution on lens
- E Build up of active protein

Answer E

Proteins from the tear film attach to contact lens surfaces within minutes of insertion. However, some time must elapse before these proteins denature and cause discomfort so they are unlikely to be the cause of an initial discomfort upon lens insertion.

Question 10.4

Which of the following should not be considered when selecting an appropriate solution system for an individual patient?
- A Lens type
- B Replacement schedule
- C Patient profile
- D Wearing modality
- E Lens power

Answer E

The power of the lens is irrelevant when deciding upon an appropriate lens care system.

Question 10.5

Soft contact lens sterilization can be achieved by:
- A Soaking in disinfection solution alone
- B Cleaning step prior to soaking in disinfection solution

- C Heat to 80°C for 20 minutes
- D Heat to 118°C for 30 minutes
- E Soaking in 3 per cent hydrogen peroxide

Answer D

Heat sterilization, though now less used, is possible after bringing the soft material up to 118°C for 30 minutes.

Question 10.6

Which of the following statements is false?
- A Denatured protein can lead to reduced lens comfort and vision
- B Active protein can cause reduced lens comfort
- C Denatured protein can cause red eye reactions
- D Protein binds to soft lens surfaces as well as entering the matrix of the lens
- E Protein-removing tablets are only effective on active proteins

Answer B

Active protein does not adversely affect comfort.

Question 10.7

Which of the following solution properties has the least effect on initial comfort?
- A Low pH
- B Viscosity
- C Tonicity
- D Preservative concentration
- E High pH

Answer B

As viscosity is linked less to the presence of ions in solution than the other options, it will have less effect on initial comfort.

Question 10.8

According to the health belief model, which of the following statements is true?
- A Compliance will be enhanced if an individual is less susceptible to developing the medical condition
- B Compliance will be enhanced if the individual believes the medical condition is not serious
- C A patient has more opportunities not to comply with a procedure, than to follow it
- D Non-compliance is more likely when there are fewer reasons not to follow instructions
- E A and C only

Answer C

The more reasons to avoid following instructions, the more likely the patient will be non-compliant. This is dealt with by the health belief model which notes that a patient has more opportunities not to comply with a procedure than to follow it appropriately.

Question 10.9

Amongst student contact lens wearers, which of the following is the least commonly practised activity?
- A Protein-removal cleaning
- B Hand-washing
- C Lens case cleaning
- D Surfactant cleaning
- E Lens disinfection

Answer C

Lens cases are a significant source of infection for the contact lens wearer and the importance of case hygiene and replacement is emphasized by an analysis of user habits.

Question 10.10

Which of the following statements is false?
- A Cleaning and rinsing together removes 99 per cent of micro-organisms
- B Multi-purpose solutions can contain cleaning and protein removing properties
- C Wetting solutions encourage an even distribution of tears over the lens on insertion
- D Soft lens cases can be safely rinsed with tap water and allowed to air dry
- E A non-wetting RGP lens can result from over-polishing during manufacture

Answer D

Studies have shown that more than 50 per cent of contact lens cases have been found to be contaminated with bacteria and 4 per cent with amoeboid species. Many of these may originate from tap water and will adhere to the case surface in a biofilm which air-drying would do little to compromise. A disinfectant should be employed and a mechanical rubbing action may be necessary to disrupt the biofilm and reduce the risk of infection.

Question 11.1

Which of the following statements regarding the closed eye environment is false?

A   Tear pH becomes more acidic
B   Tear osmolarity decreases
C   Available oxygen decreases
D   Corneal demands for oxygen decreases
E   Lens temperature increases

Answer D
Corneal metabolism continues in the closed lid state and a decrease in oxygen demand is not found.

Question 11.2
The critical average transmissibility to allow 4 per cent or less overnight oedema is?
A   34.3
B   87.0
C   24.1
D   120.0
E   67.4

Answer B
The critical corneal oxygen requirement to allow less than or equal to 4 per cent oedema is stated as a Dk/t average of 87 at 20°C.

Question 11.3
During normal closed eye sleep (i.e. without contact lens wear) the cornea swells by an average of:
A   0 per cent
B   2 per cent
C   4 per cent
D   8 per cent
E   20 per cent

Answer C
Four per cent is the average closed eye swelling for the non-lens wearing eye.

Question 11.4
Which of the following signs in a daily contact lens wearer would not contraindicate switching to extended wear?
A   Corneal staining
B   >grade 1 bulbar conjunctival hyperaemia
C   Corneal oedema
D   >grade 1 palpebral papillae redness
E   Small, non-staining corneal scar

Answer E
A small non-staining scar should have no effect upon the successful wear of extended wear lenses. All the other options could hinder comfort or corneal metabolism.

Question 11.5
Which of the following instruments cannot be used to observe and/or measure significant amounts of corneal oedema?
A   Optical pachometer
B   Slit-lamp biomicroscope
C   Tearscope
D   Ultrasonic pachometer
E   Keratometer

Answer C
Whereas all the other options allow visualization of some aspect of the cornea, a tearscope will only give information relating to the tear film so would not usefully allow observation of corneal oedema.

Question 11.6
Which fitting and aftercare schedule is recommended for extended wear patients?
A   1 week DW/1 night EW/1 week review/3 month routine
B   1 week EW/4 week review/3 month routine
C   1 night EW/1 week review/6 month routine
D   1week DW/1 night EW/1 week review/6 month routine
E   1 week DW/1 week EW/3 month routine

Answer A
A short period of daily wear is highly recommended to assess the response to the lens fit and material. An assessment after the first night may elicit information as to the patient's adaptation to extended wear, and a long-term three month aftercare regime is advisable to allow accurate detection of any potential long-term reaction to extended wear.

Question 11.7
Which of the following observations would be made in the presence of 6 per cent corneal oedema due to soft lens wear?
A   Central corneal clouding
B   Two folds
C   Two striae
D   Significantly reduced visual acuity
E   Five striae

Answer C
During a critical assessment of corneal oedema, one to three striae may indicate a 5–7 per cent oedematous response.

Question 11.8
Which of the following conditions is less likely to be observed with silicone hydrogel materials when compared to hydrogel lenses?
A   SEAL lesions
B   'Mucin balls'
C   Corneal oedema
D   Infiltrates
E   CLARE

Answer C
Corneal oedema is less likely with the silicone hydrogel materials as they have excellent oxygen transmission to help avoid this.

Question 11.9
Appropriate management approach for CLPU is:
A   Loosen fit
B   Increase oxygen supply
C   Change solution regime
D   Cease lens wear, monitor and refer if signs/symptoms increase
E   Refer immediately

Answer D
Cessation of lens wear is a sensible approach to remove the potential source of the ulceration and to allow healing to occur. Careful monitoring of the patient is needed to ensure that this healing does take place and to look for any indications of infective activity that might warrant medical intervention.

Question 11.10
Appropriate management for suspected infectious ulcer is?
A   Remove lens and allow to resolve
B   Refer immediately
C   Refit and increase oxygen supply
D   Use ocular lubricants
E   Change solution regimen

Answer B
Many pathogens involved in an active microbial keratitis may lead to significant inflammatory response and corneal scarring in a matter of hours and so in the event of a suspected infectious ulcer, immediate referral is appropriate.

Question 12.1
Which of the following is generally not a primary function of therapeutic lenses?
A   Pain relief
B   Correcting ametropia
C   Promoting epithelial healing

D Sealing corneal perforations
E Improving visual acuity in distorted corneas

Answer B
The main functions of the lens are protective and prophylactic, irrespective of any refractive error. This is not to say that refractive correction cannot be incorporated into such lenses, but it is not usually their primary function.

Question 12.2
Rigid contact lenses are useful in therapeutic lens fitting because they:
A Are more comfortable
B Allow greater tear exchange
C Are fitted with smaller total diameters
D Form a liquid tear lens and smooth refracting surface
E Have higher oxygen transmissibility

Answer D
The RGP lens provides a smooth refracting surface over the top of the liquid tear lens so significantly improving the visual potential of any cornea that has been compromised. This would be the case with, for example, keratoconus, epithelial dystrophies and iatrogenic or traumatic corneal scarring.

Question 12.3
Which of the following is not an indication for therapeutic lens wear?
A Bullous keratopathy
B Filamentary keratitis
C Meibomian gland dysfunction
D Exposure keratitis
E Recurrent erosion

Answer C
Meibomian gland dysfunction is often described as posterior blepharitis and is managed in a similar way to blepharitis. Issues of lid hygiene are important and lid massaging and warm compresses give relief. If an infective component is isolated then an antibacterial agent may be introduced and, occasionally, an anti-inflammatory may be considered, particularly to alleviate any secondary inflammatory responses. Unlike the other four options, contact lenses are not advised in the management of this condition.

Question 12.4
Which lens type would be least appropriate for management of exposure keratitis?

A Rigid gas-permeable
B Scleral
C Hydrogel
D Silicone rubber
E Silicone hydrogel

Answer A
Obviously the appropriate management of exposure keratopathy must address the reduction of corneal exposure. A rigid gas-permeable lens will still allow exposure of a large peripheral area of cornea. All the other options will allow full corneal coverage and hence reduce the adverse corneal response.

Question 12.5
Potential toxicity effects can be minimized while topical medication is being used concurrently with soft lenses by using:
A Preserved drops
B Daily disposable lenses
C High-water content materials
D Smaller diameter lenses
E Thinner lens designs

Answer B
The use of preserved topical medication with soft lenses *in situ* is always a concern due to the introduced molecules being retained within the lens material so prolonging exposure to potentially toxic substances. This effect may be minimized by the use of non-preserved single dose drug units. Concerns with regard to prolonged exposure to the drug itself may be somewhat alleviated by the use of regular replacement lenses. The balance of the cost with safe management usually leads to a weekly replacement regime being established.

Question 12.6
Which of the following is not a prerequisite for successful therapeutic lens fitting?
A Individual practitioner management
B Easy access to clinics
C Careful case selection
D Realistic patient expectations
E Adequate patient selection

Answer A
Patients often state a preference for individual practitioner management, but it is rarely, if ever, essential and systems of shared management combined with clear and effective patient instruction allow far more efficient and useful deployment of the practitioner's time. All the other stated

options have a direct impact upon the success of therapeutic lens wear.

Question 12.7
Soft 'bandage lenses' used in therapeutic lens fitting can vary in total diameter from:
A 14.0 mm to 15.0 mm
B 9.0 mm to 12.0 mm
C 14.0 mm to 20.0 mm
D 8.0 mm to 11.0 mm
E 13.0 mm to 15.0 mm

Answer C
As good corneal coverage is so often essential in bandage lens use, larger diameters tend to be useful.

Question 12.8
Which of the following is a less critical requirement of a soft therapeutic lens?
A High oxygen transmissibility
B Choice of total diameters
C Parameter stability
D Large power range
E Economical

Answer D
As stated earlier, while refractive correction is a useful facility, it is not the main reason for using bandage lenses so a wide power range is less critical.

Question 12.9
During aftercare of an extended wear bandage lens fit, which of the following may not be necessary?
A Assessment of lens fit
B Visual acuity measurement
C Slit-lamp examination
D Assessment of tissue healing
E Lens removal

Answer E
Lens removal may not be necessary providing there is an adequate view of the relevant ocular structures and there is no indication for changing or improving the lens.

Question 12.10
When using rose bengal stain, which of the following statements is false?
A Can result in significant discomfort for the patient
B Can stain lids and skin surrounding the eye
C Tissue staining is best observed under blue light
D Stains dead tissue red

E   The tiniest amount possible should be instilled

Answer C

Rose bengal is a true stain and does not fluoresce. It does not require a particular wavelength in order to be activated and the best view of stained tissue is gained under white light.

Index